VITALITY

HOW TO CREATE THE LIFE
& BODY YOU WANT.
A SMART SAVVY LIFESTYLE
GUIDE FOR SUPER BUSY PEOPLE.

NIKKI FOGDEN-MOORE

You may not, under any circumstances, print, reproduce or use any portion of this book for public or commercial purposes without written permission from the author.

You may not, under any circumstances, print or reproduce any or all of this book and attach another name to it

The author has strived to be as accurate and complete as possible in creating this book, however, assumes no responsibility for errors, omissions, or contrary interpretation of the content herein.

This book is not intended for use as a complete source of health and wellbeing advice. Readers are advised to seek services of qualified, medical professionals or health and nutrition experts concerning any health concerns you may have, or for specific advice relating to your own situation.

Thanks for reading... And enjoy!

Second Edition 2019
ISBN-13: 978-0-6482618-3-4

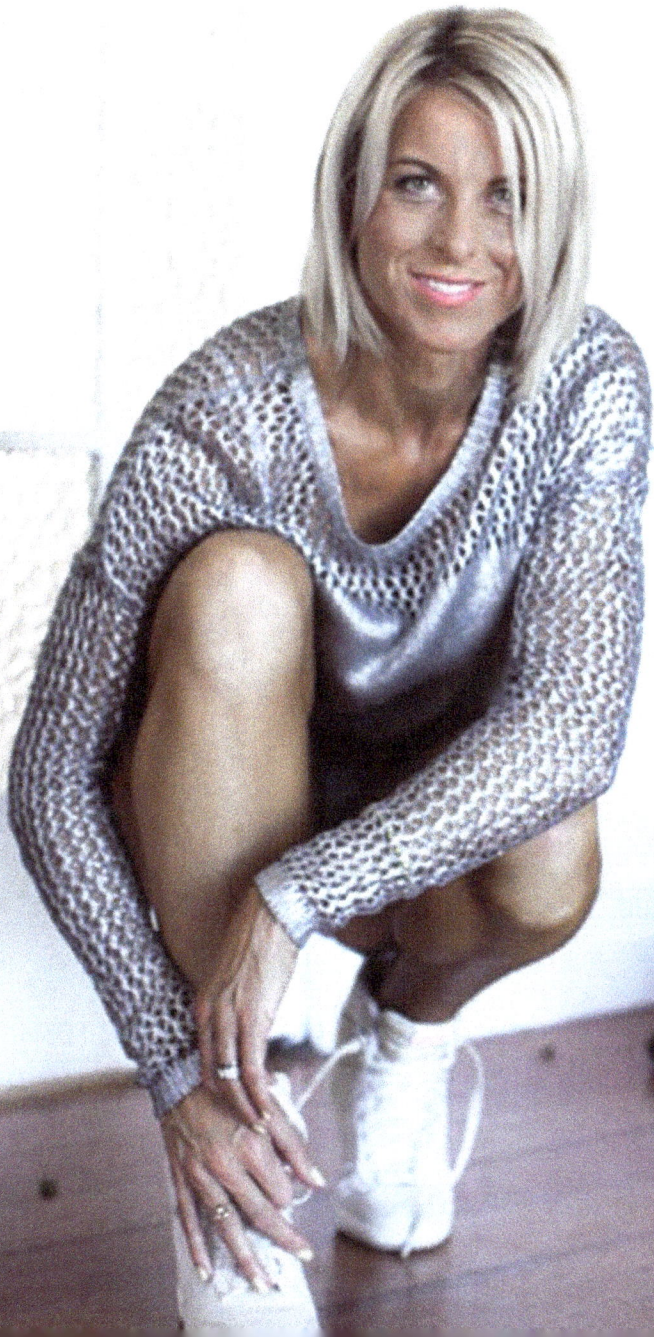

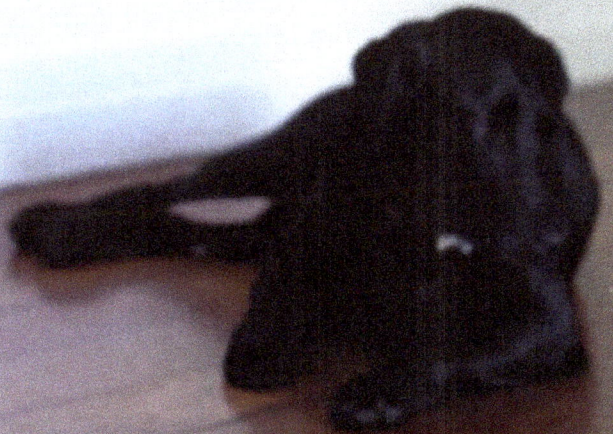

CONTENTS

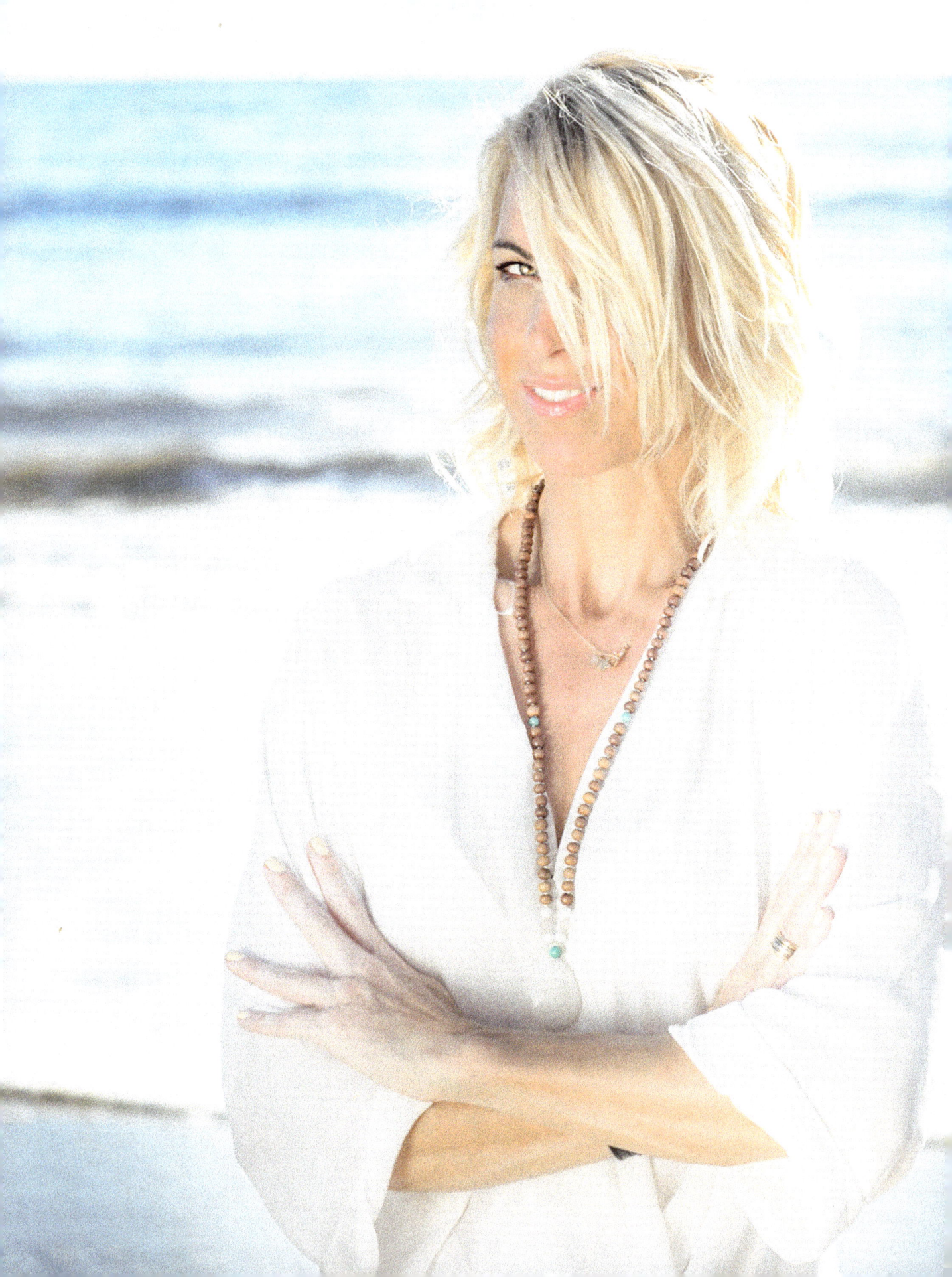

What is Vitality?

Jumping out of bed with energy
Feeling fantastic, inside and out
Feeling empowered, not restricted, by your body
Being connected to every cell in your body
Mental and physical balance

Vitality is strength, flexibility, agility and power – it's how you feel not how you look.

It's being connected, having respect for your body and appreciating the now.

It's knowing you can use nature as your gym and that you are capable of whatever you put your mind to. Vitality is my reason for being, it motivates me to think outside the box, to train as I feel and enjoy the benefits of fresh air and a fresh perspective.

Vitality is about being your personal best, which means that you can create the life that you want. What does Vitality mean to you?

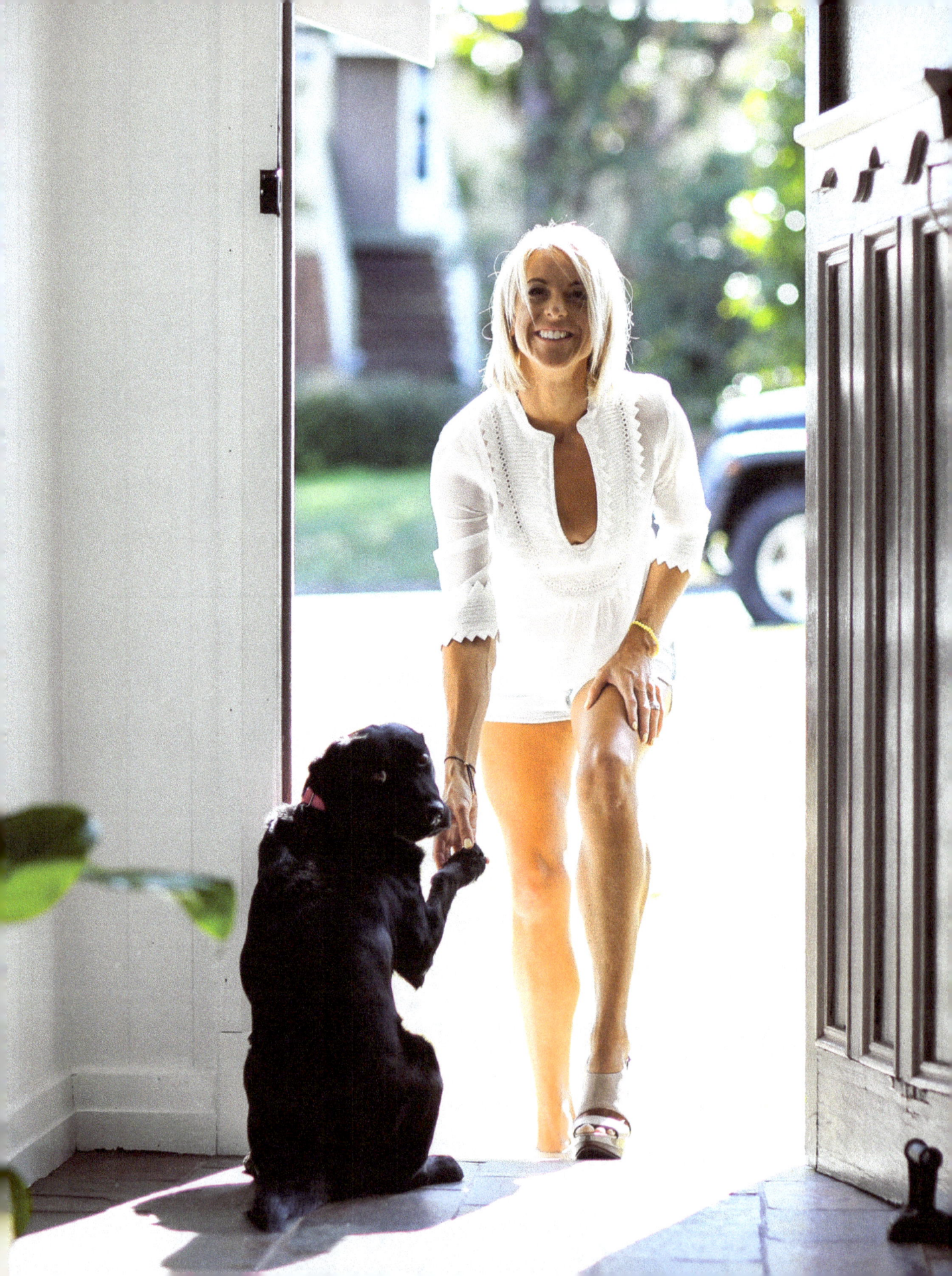

Welcome to feeling fantastic!

Welcome! I am so excited to be able to help you gently yet powerfully transition your lifestyle, to make this THE year you evolve your health and fitness life!

I'll be sharing plenty of tips, strategies, tools and advice on the following pages, but I want to let you in on a secret upfront: they're all born out of one guiding principle.

The key to achieving your health goals always comes back to the most simple, yet most important rule of all: ACTIVE LIVING.

But before we dive in, I need to ask... are you:
A) A person that DOES things with life? or
B) A person that LIFE does things to?

You need to really BELIEVE in the answer...

Let's assume if you're still reading that this is going to be about type A – doing things with life. No more excuses, no more procrastination – whatever it takes, you're prepared to do it.

If this is the case, then you need to remind yourself that every day counts and every day is a gift. This is also a good time to consider why your health is important to you, and what do you really believe its value is?

What is active living?
- ★ Moving more in your daily life
- ★ Always prioritising the active option
- ★ Shaking up your sedentary rut

In these pages, we'll cover everything from simple fitness routines you can easily incorporate into your day, to ways you can keep your family inspired, to tips for achieving balance on those busy days that demand every last shred of patience!

In our increasingly busy, over-scheduled, often sedentary lives, we regularly feel we're "too busy" to find time for structured exercise programs. I understand the feeling, which is why I believe you need to create routines and habits that suit your lifestyle. In that sense, everything can be tied back to my central philosophy of active living.

My goal: is to inspire you to enjoy fresh food through delicious and simple recipes, while giving you an improved knowledge of nutrition that gets back to basics – along with a real set of tools for fitness that can be easily integrated into your life.

Your role: is to take responsibility and commit to the process of improving your lifestyle with healthier, more active routines. This is a 'no excuses' book; the aim of the game is to recalibrate your day-to-day life around an active lifestyle. I want you to learn how to define your personal best, to be empowered to make great decisions, and to create the life you truly want.

Why should you listen to me?

I'm not just planning to tell you how to do it – I'm actually going to show you how.
After 15 years of coaching clients on how to integrate health and exercise into everyday life, I've come to the conclusion that there is no 'one-size-fits all' solution for every person. We all face similar challenges when it comes to prioritising our health, but the road towards a more active and healthier lifestyle is different for every person.

That said, I believe that maintaining your health is not about sticking to strict exercise regimes or gruelling workouts. It's not about limiting your diet and subsisting on protein shakes and low-calorie meals.

It's much simpler than that. I believe it's about rebooting your hard drive and adopting new ways of achieving old tasks, so you can get the best out of your day.

My clients don't need me anymore, which is exactly how I like it. That is my goal: to empower people to make their own way. I want to inspire you to reach your potential, engage you to think differently about food and fitness and empower you to put all of this together and make your health and fitness goals a reality. All of this, without having to turn your life upside down. I'm telling you, it can be done!

The ingredients for feeling fantastic are really the same for everyone; they all come back to the three key pillars for Vitality:

FRESH AIR

FRESH FOOD

FRESH PERSPECTIVE

The simple, effective strategies I share in this book – and on my website, in my podcasts and via my newsletter – are all based around these central pillars. They help me think clearer, make better decisions and generally be more productive, whether I'm writing, training, coaching or managing my day-to-day life.

I hope I can inspire and guide you to get your goals off paper and into real life by sharing these simple steps. A goal does not become a reality until you create action. To BE something, you must DO something.

And the secret to having your best body ever is really no secret at all; it simply means living a healthy lifestyle, making it a part of your life. It may sound daunting, but don't worry; I'm going to show you how it's done.

Welcome to feeling fantastic!

Health & Happiness

Nikki x

P.S. I'VE CHANGED THE ORDER OF THE PILLARS TO KICKSTART WITH A FRESH PERSPECTIVE – IN MY EXPERIENCE, I'VE FOUND THAT NOTHING WILL ALIGN UNTIL YOU TRULY HAVE A SENSE OF SELF-BELIEF AND CONVICTION TO LOOK AND FEEL YOUR PERSONAL BEST ON A SUBCONSCIOUS LEVEL.

Dedication

To Ann, Trevor, Kiki, Spook, Roxy Dog and my crazy family, who never seem to stay in one place for long – thank you for having a zest for life and for giving me the belief that we can create the life we want

I've always believed that to truly achieve your personal best and appreciate everything that life offers, you need to have the right people around you: those who share your passion for making a difference, who stand out in the crowd and have carved a personal niche in what they do.

Whether it's on a local or global scale, the following people have been part of this process and my journey bringing VITALITY to life. So here's a very special shout out to: Keith Hamlyn, Ashley Streff, Sam Frysteen and Stu Gibson for their stunning photography; Layne and Kirk, who have always made sure the guest room was ready and are like family; Ben Wilson for introducing me to Namotu and being great to work with over the years. Renata, Janine, Kylie and the LBD Group ladies, for a sense of community where craziness is the norm; to Greg, Nathan and the team from Body Science; Christine Barry, Tara Wolf, Rebecca and the team from *Women's Health & Fitness Magazine*, Neil and The Outrigger Resorts and a very special mention to Richard Molnar. In memory too of Chris Drake and family – always remember to "Smile Like Drake".

I'd like to thank Team Vitality - Sasha, Alina and all the trainers along the way that share the vision for philosophy that Life is a Gym. Sarah (my editor who had to review 40,000 words…!) and Claire, my talented book cover designer. You are all fabulous.

To some of my very first clients, who over a decade ago who joined me on my retreats, attended my corporate workshops and those I coached one to one, to the amazing CEOs and industry leaders I work with today who are creating real business vitality with a fresh perspective for all levels within their corporations. Thank you for wanting to be your best and elevate all you are doing – you all rock!

How to use this book

This book is designed to be picked up often…

★ For you to write notes in
★ For you to scribble in the margin
★ For you to photograph a page that resonates and save it on your phone
★ For you to use sticky notes and pull out pages if you want!

In a nutshell, I want you to think of this book as a portable tool for fitness, food and fitspiration. It's designed for busy people – because honestly, who's not busy these days? – and all of the key worksheets shared throughout are also available as printable PDFs on a dedicated webpage, along with a virtual support network complete with videos, podcasts and extra tips and tools.

Most importantly, as you read this I want you to think about how you can ACTUALLY create the life, and as a result, the body, you want. I want you to learn and apply some of the things you read, so that they turn into habits and become a seamless part of your daily life.

I trust that as you read this book, you can imagine me sitting with you (I hope that's okay!) and supporting you as your coach. And I hope that when you stop and make a choice, you might think about the options available to you and select the one that the healthy, happy, fit version of you would choose.

Okay, are you ready to get started? Imagine you're a computer and a new operating system has been released: it's time to re-wire your hard drive so you can perform at your peak. So throw out the usual procrastinations, because now is your moment to start **living the life your future you will thank you for.**

What are you waiting for…? Let's get started!

You only have one body – so why risk your long-term health by living a sedentary, inactive lifestyle? Read on and learn how easy it is for you to reconnect and make the most of the one body you've got, for optimal health, energy and vitality, now and as you age.

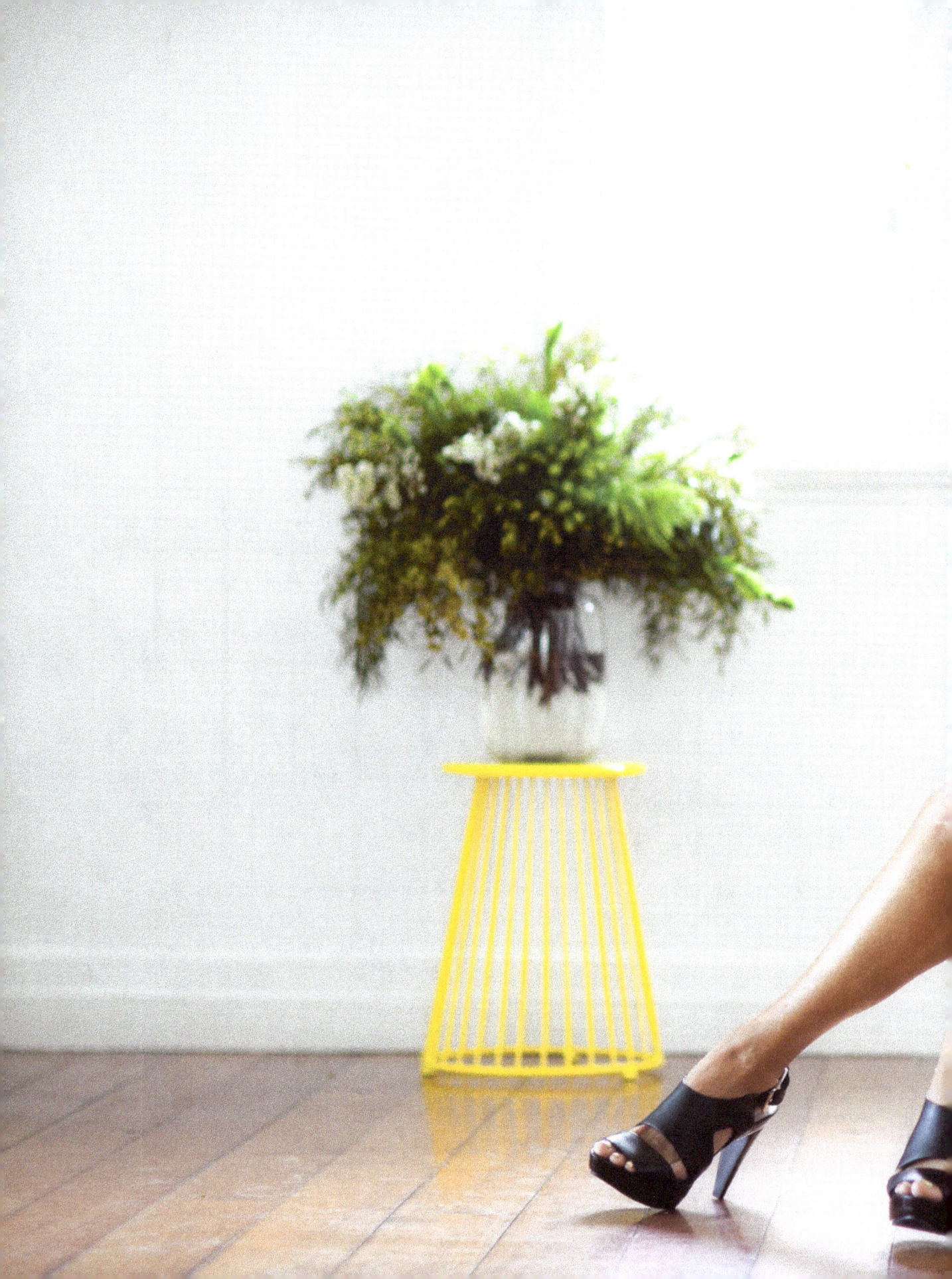

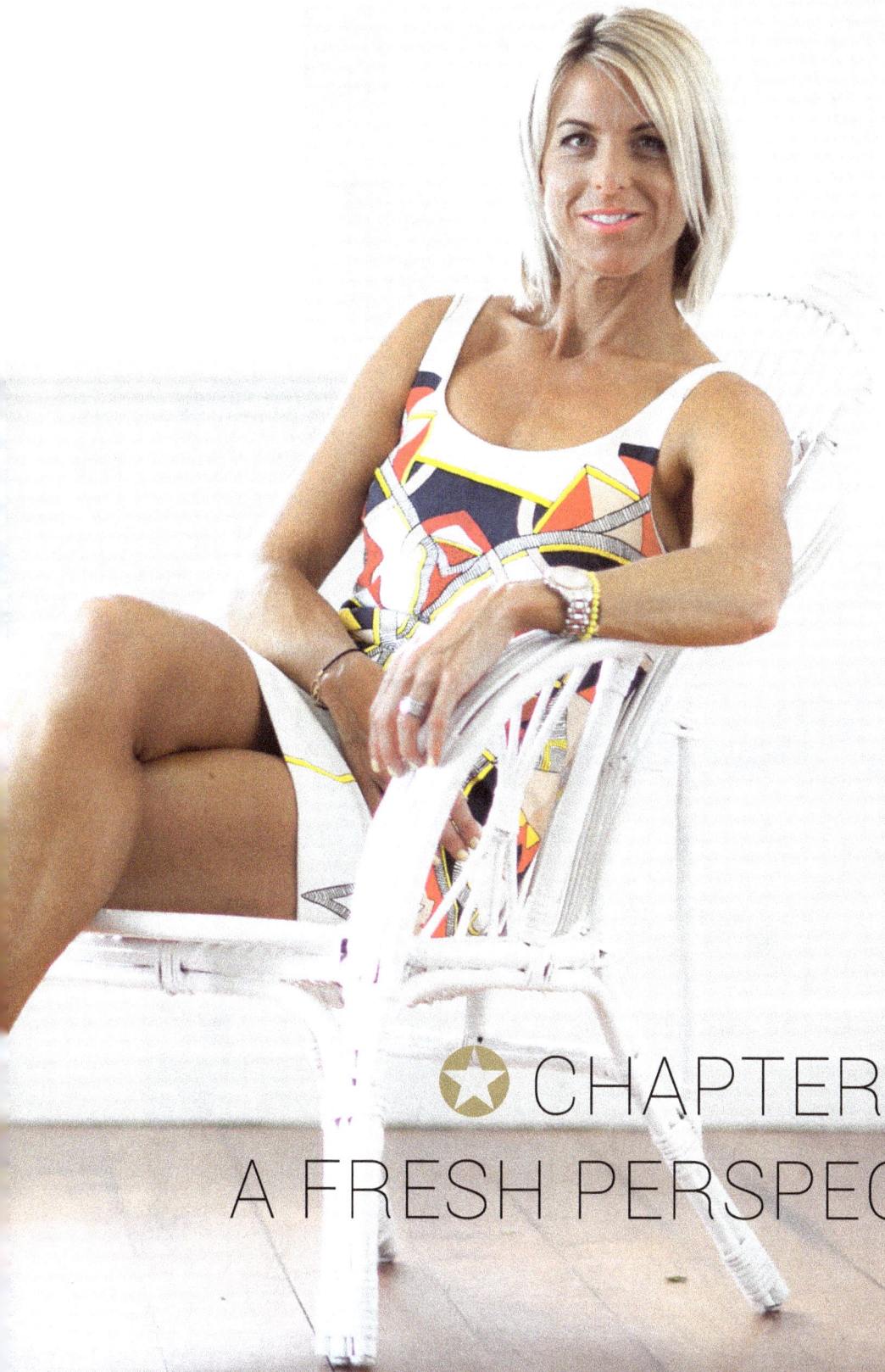

★ CHAPTER ONE:
A FRESH PERSPECTIVE

LIFE HAS NO REMOTE
GET UP & CHANGE IT
YOURSELF

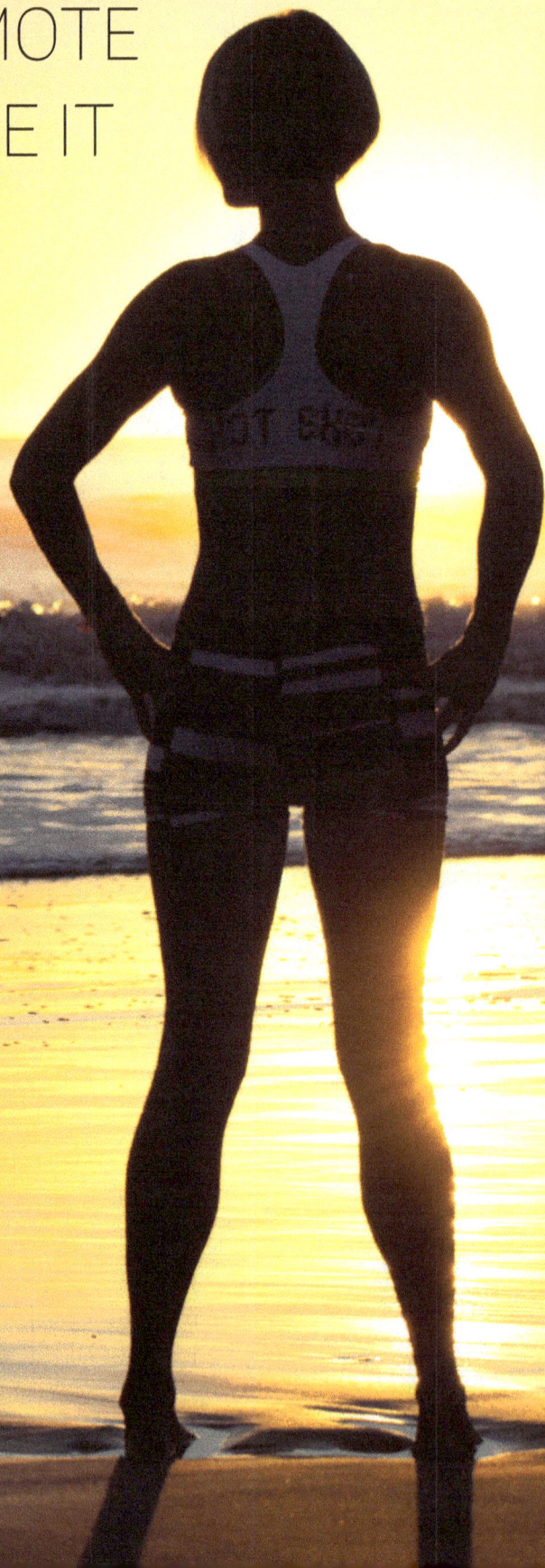

Reclaiming your mojo

After 12 years of coaching I told our team the other day we specialise in mojos.

We help people look and feel their personal best, and teach them how to keep it that way, which is a fancy way of saying that we help people get their mojo back.

That has been my absolute mission since founding Life's a Gym and it's one of the best ways I can think of to sum up this book!

Sometimes, life just takes over and stops you from living. You may look up one day and realise 15 years have flown by. You have the high profile job title, the corner office, and a wonderful family. You may even have the latest computers and gadgets, amazing pairs of designer shoes, incredible travel photos of overseas adventures and a home you're proud of.

But still, something is missing.

You're not looking in the mirror thinking, **'Damn, I look good. And I feel great!'**

Maybe along the way, while you were building your empire, kicking goals in your career, being an "A" grade parent or a wonderful, supportive partner...

Maybe, you lost your mojo?

Well, I'm going to let you in on a few of my personal tips to show you how you can get your MOJO BACK!

What is Mojo?

Dictionary Term: mojo

Noun

  // A magic charm, talisman, or spell.
  // Magic power.

Most commonly, we hear mojo referred to as that special spark that someone has – that inner vibe, connection, glow and "can do" approach.

According to Wikipedia, mojo means "finding the magic in what we do". To have "lost your mojo" refers to a loss of inspiration or creative genius; a loss of that special spark

I think my Niktionary definition explains it best:

"Mojo is a special positive force of amazingness that means you are operating at your personal best in all things mental, emotional, spiritual and physical."

Now, who wouldn't want a bit of that?

Get Your Health & Fitness Mojo Back — FOR GOOD

Step 1. Give yourself permission to be absolutely happy.
This is essential! Those who love you want you to shine in all your glory, simply for being the person you are. Once you understand that achieving your own happiness is not only possible, but it's absolutely crucial if you want to be able to enjoy your life and give back to others, you'll realise that you don't have to keep putting yourself last on the list

What is preventing you from prioritising your own goals?
Time – Money – Experience – Know-how – Training – Babysitters – Energy – Willpower – Commitment – Support – Drive – Motivation – Discipline

Step 2: Discover what makes your heart sing.
When was the last time you did something that made you smile or feel like a kid inside again? It could be as simple as diving into the ocean, bouncing on a trampoline, catching up with close friends that you laugh with like nobody else, playing music that made you want to dance around the room or going for a run. Whatever it is, you must figure out what you enjoy doing.

Step 3: Start doing the things you love more often.
Avoid apologising for making a new schedule or reshuffling a few things in your life if it's going to give you more time to do the things that make your heart sing. This is your mojo we are talking about here! Create actions and behaviour changes that reflect where you want to be – not what you want to avoid.

YOU'RE NEVER
TOO OLD FOR
HANDSTANDS

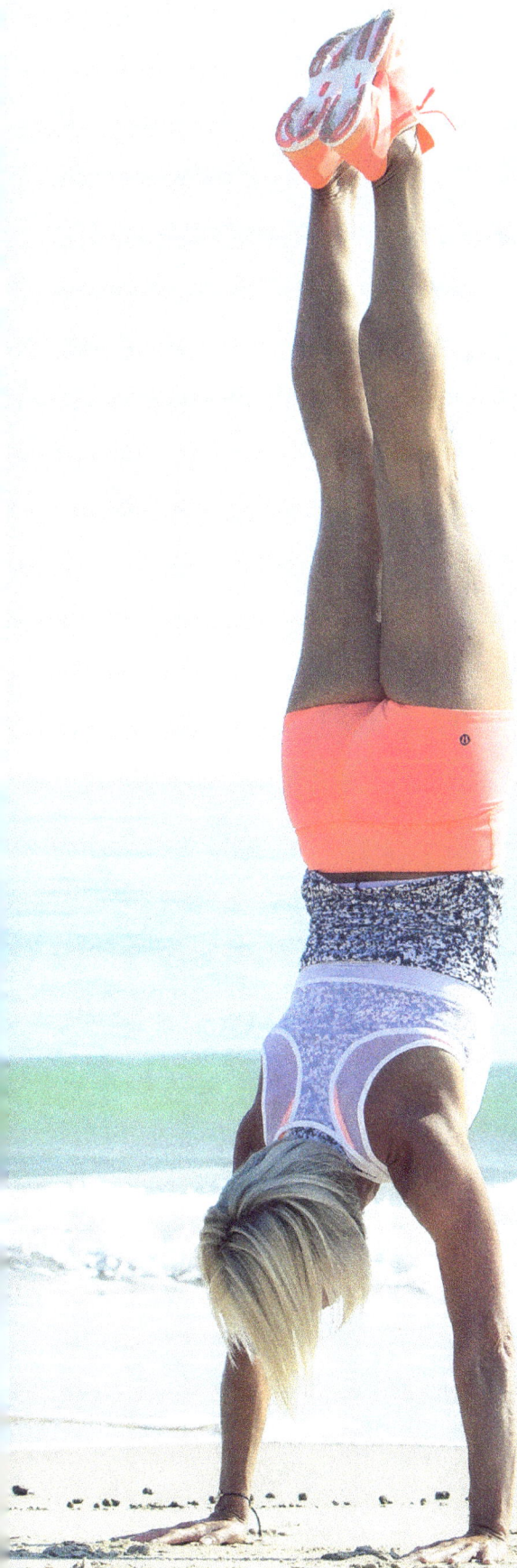

Step 4: Believe to achieve.

Getting your mojo back must be done with pure conviction. This conviction to act must come from within; you cannot be swayed by the opinions of others. This is your life and your mojo! If you need to work out why you have been denying yourself happiness, then take some time to read, learn and register your common habits and reactions to situations.

Step 5: Ask for help.

Once you've established that it's time to find your mojo again, go and ask for some help. It doesn't need to be a professional coach; you could start by signing your friends and family up to do something fun, re-writing your personal goals and aspirations, or leading by example in your workplace to encourage others to put their health first.

And always, always remember: It's never too late to be the fittest, healthiest version of you. Every day, every meal, every moment is a new opportunity to make smart choices.

Healthy Mind, Healthy Body

The two go hand-in-hand.

If you're lacking results with your fitness or health goals, then maybe it's time to test how serious you actually are about your personal health and wellbeing by setting yourself a personal challenge.

Our subconscious plays a huge role in the patterns we follow in achieving happiness and success. If you don't have a real, deep down belief that being fit and healthy is important to you, then you will never truly reach those goals.

You also need to feel the pain of not reaching those goals. For many people, they avoid the opportunities to feel this pain by shifting the goal posts; when they're carrying extra weight, for instance, they avoid the mirror, skulk out of the frame when photos are being taken and buy looser clothing the next size up.

If you're okay with living in this unsatisfied state, and you're not prepared to make some sacrifices in order to create a healthier, slimmer, energetic and vital lifestyle, then the truth is, you'll never claw your way out of it.

BE TRUE
TO WHO
YOU ARE

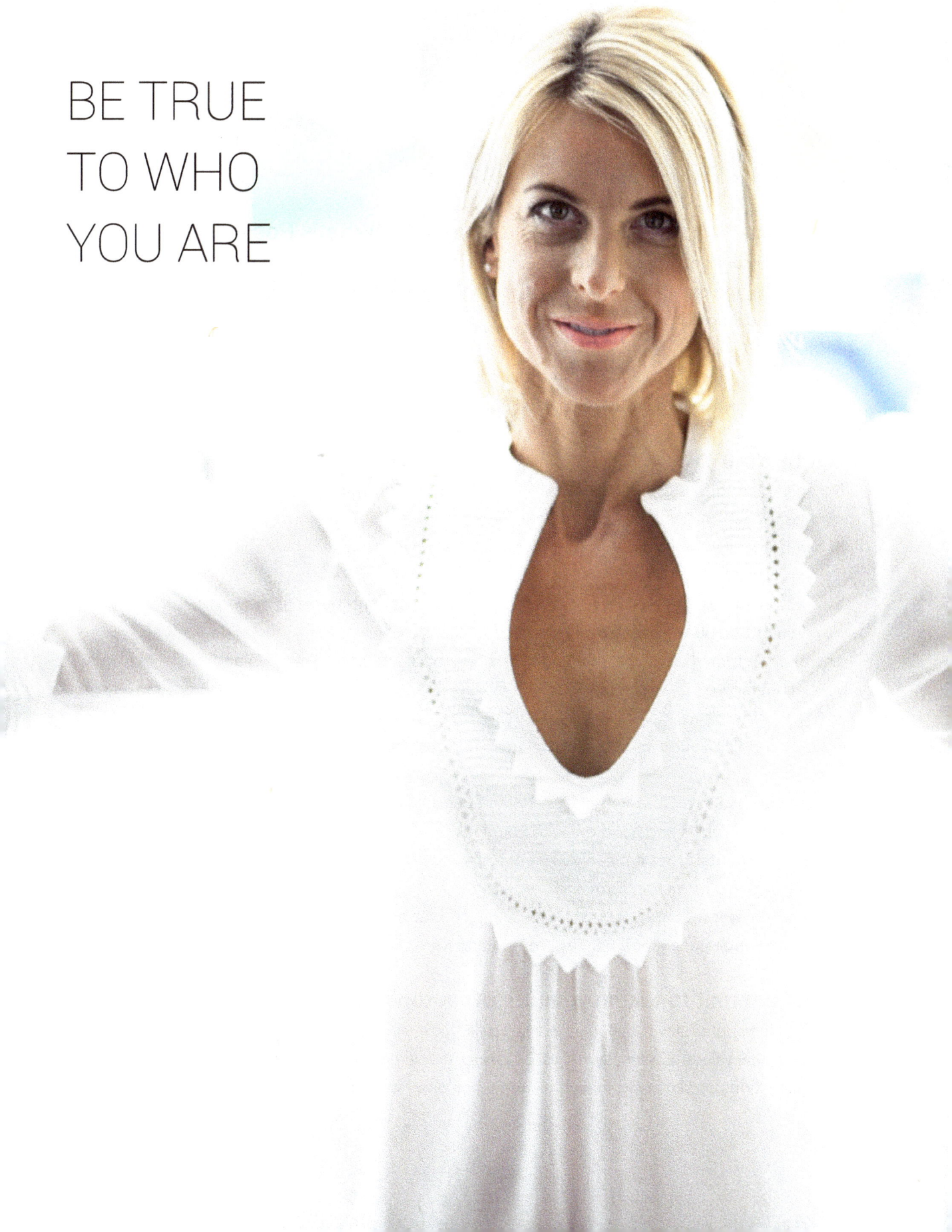

Being in the best shape of your life takes **total conviction** that you deserve to be healthy, that you want to be healthy and that you're prepared to go after it, no matter the cost.

Age is no barrier. Your mindset is.

Turn Your "Impossible" Into The Question: "What's Possible"?

It absolutely does not matter what age, shape or fitness level you are, nor does it matter what your goal is. You can always improve and reach your personal best with some straightforward thinking and a no-nonsense approach.

So how can you find truly authentic reasons to start putting your health and fitness goals at the top of your agenda and ensure they become a deep-set belief as an important part of your life?

Define Your Why

My absolute motto is 'Create the Life You Want'. Connecting to your purpose will be your anchor, your conviction and your true north for achieving your goals. The simple truth is, until your goals and your true self-belief align, you won't achieve what you want.

Every morning, we get a chance to create a new day that contributes to our goals, our vision, our dreams and our wishes. If a key area in your life is to be fit and healthy and to achieve your personal best, then it's crucial that you take a step back and start accepting and loving the body you've been given.

Start by creating your own definition of what «the best shape of your life» means.

Active and healthy: Does it mean just being fit and healthy enough to prevent illness, enjoy day- to-day activities and hang out with your kids?
Testing the limits: Does it mean you want to test the limits of your physical potential and bring out the best in your shape, form and flexibility?
Athletic prowess: Or do you want to take it a step further and see what your body is capable of in terms of appearance, endurance, strength and performance?

Then: commit to taking your life off autopilot.

Taking full responsibility for yourself is a key pillar for my coaching with clients and is part of my own personal values. Essentially, it's about taking your life off autopilot and becoming accountable for your actions and knowing that you – and you alone – create the life you want.

Being informed and educated on how you can truly reach your potential and live a happy, fulfilling life starts with taking responsibility. There are no quick fixes. But the journey towards conquering your health goals all begins in your mindset.

"If you don't create the life you want, you will get the one you're given".

I'm not sure who wrote that quote, but I saw it almost 20 years ago and it s been the backbone of anything I ve done ever since then. I'm not saying it s been plain sailing, or that I don't constantly make mistakes and need to course-correct! I do take full responsibility for where I am now and the journey so far.

Are you living up to your true potential and creating a lifestyle that enables everything you desire to be possible… Or are you still just wishing and thinking about it?

How do you create the life you want?

Visualise the future 'you' and start actively living it. Here s how: Take a pen and paper and write down what you look FORWARD to as the future you. Be honest, open and specific when you write answers to these questions:

What does the best of you do:

What time do you get up?

_____

What's your job?

_____

How do you workout?

_____

What do you wear?

_____

Where does future you live and what is your lifestyle like?

_____

What does future you do for fun?

_____

What does the best, most healthy you eat?

_____

How does the healthy you stay fit and happy?

_____

What exercises and activities make you smile?

_____

Who does the best, healthy, happy you spend their time with?

_____

How does the healthy, happy and successful you stay motivated and overcome challenges?

_____

Take a look at your list and highlight all the things you could start doing NOW.

And start living the list above – why wait for an enormous life event to get you moving towards creating the life you really want to be living?

Keep this list front and centre. Live the life you want now by implementing small, daily changes that benefit the best of you. You ll be surprised how easy it is to shed off excuses when you start with small steps that create lasting change.

As George Bernard Shaw says, "Life is not about finding yourself, but creating yourself."

BRAINSTORM WHY BEING HEALTHY IS IMPORTANT TO YOU

e.g. To run around and play with my kids
So I can stop catching the flu and feeling under the weather
To jump out of bed with energy in the morning
Energy, vitality, stamina, strength, health, fitness, active, electric

Reality check: For many people the negative body image and lack of self-acceptance starts as young as 10 or 12 and carries through until they hit retirement age. Some people are confronted with an illness or accident that puts everything in a "new perspective".

Why wait for that to happen and ignore one of most important aspects of inner peace and balance?

So, you've found your why:
Let's move on to setting your goals...

Believe = Achieve

Whether you're part of a multinational company, work from home as an entrepreneur, are studying hard as a student or you re a full-time, at-home parent – you have a 'workplace . It is important to factor your workplace into your personal wellbeing goals, because it's the only way they can be seamlessly integrated into all aspects of your daily life.

Healthy is a lifestyle, not a chore or a side note. And achieving your health and fitness goals isn't nearly as intimidating or impossible as you may think. Start getting them off paper and into action with these three key steps:

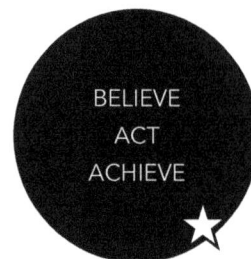

BELIEVE
ACT
ACHIEVE

1. BELIEVE: SET YOUR GOAL
Be clear about what you want to achieve and your personal mantra. This does not mean you have to shout from the rooftops and convert others. It does mean that you must feel centred and driven by this goal, for it to be sustainable. Self-belief is paramount. YES YOU CAN!

2. ACT: DEFINE THE ACTIONS REQUIRED
Hopefully by now, you can you articulate the 'why'. There is no need to justify your goal to others, but it is essential for you to be clear on why you're doing what you're doing, as it becomes a more authentic process. If you are taking steps towards your goals by tangible 'actions', then you are also showing your commitment to the end result.

3. ACHIEVE: COMMIT TO YOUR DAILY TASKS
Incremental daily steps are the secret to creating lasting change. Grand gestures and a thousand sticky notes might create a lot of noise, but they often result in no action. Quietly go about achieving your daily milestones and don't give up.

Once you feel comfortable with these three concepts, pick up a pen and a big sheet of paper. Your goals can be framed within a year, a month or a week: it s your life and the ball is in your court!

MORNING
YOUR DAY IS READY
DIVE RIGHT IN

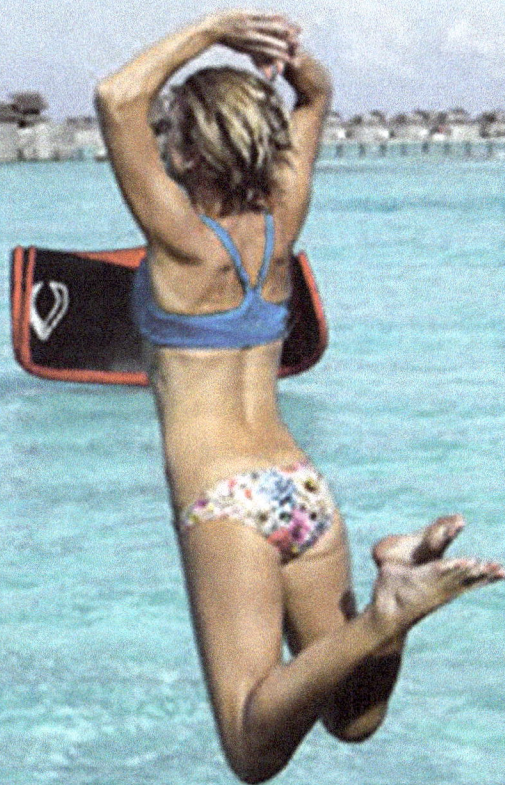

STEP 1: "MY GOALS" (WHAT YOU BELIEVE IN):
Write 1 to 5 of THE MOST IMPORTANT things you want to achieve this year. They must be:
- ★ Authentically YOU
- ★ Relevant to YOU
- ★ Meaningful to YOU

Next to each goal, write a sentence or just a few highlight words on the **WHY.** Think about all your usual goals (lose weight, start my own business, get a promotion, run a marathon race, cook at home more regularly) and consider why these didn't work? Remember – be more specific!

Goals are personal.

They can be simple, they can be grand or they can be shared. There are no rules. The art is to stop thinking about what you want and get out there and make it happen.

STEP 2: "MY ACTIONS" (WHAT YOU NEED TO DO TO MAKE IT HAPPEN):
Write the steps you need to take to get this goal off paper and into your life – from right now to ongoing. Once you have this action list then go back to the three pillars to integrate your personal goals into everyday living as daily tasks. Note, there is nothing in between – no procrastinations, no waiting for Monday, no 'I need this first'. It goes straight from goal to starting action with little steps.

STEP 3: "MY TASKS" (MILESTONE ACHIEVEMENTS TO ENSURE SUCCESS):
Now that you have your action list, you need to break these down into daily tasks. Create small steps that are easily achievable and inch you one step closer to the bigger picture. For example, healthy eating can mean going to a farmers market for fresh vegetables. If your goal is to run a 5km race, then your daily task could be getting out the door for a 20-minute walk to build up your fitness. Start with small steps to work towards creating the big change you want to see.

Setting your goals worksheet

Immediate (the next 7 days)

Short term (the next month)

Mid term (the next 6 months)

Long term (the next year +)

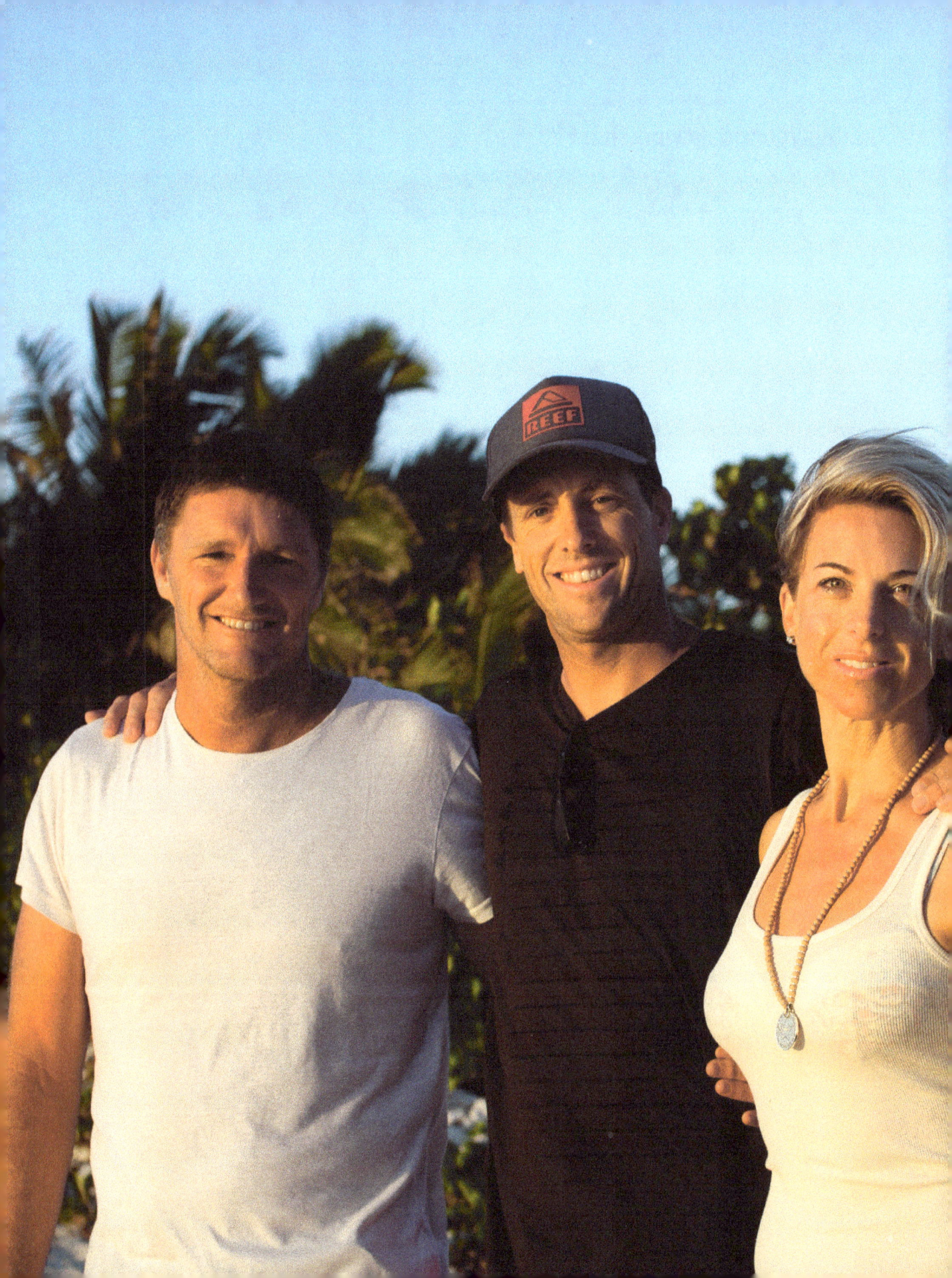

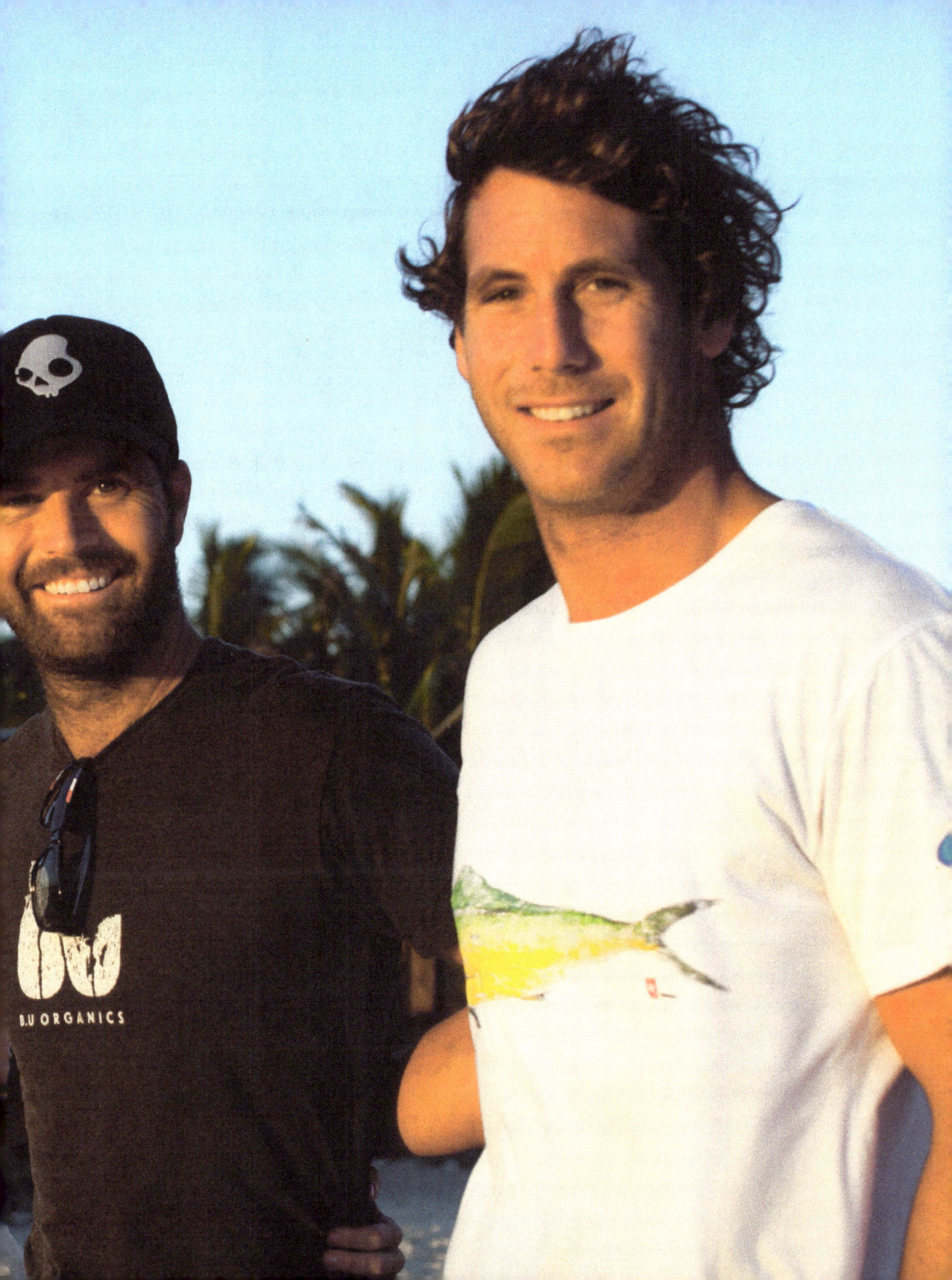

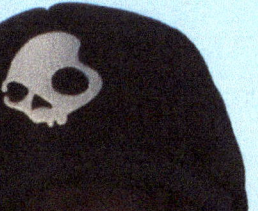

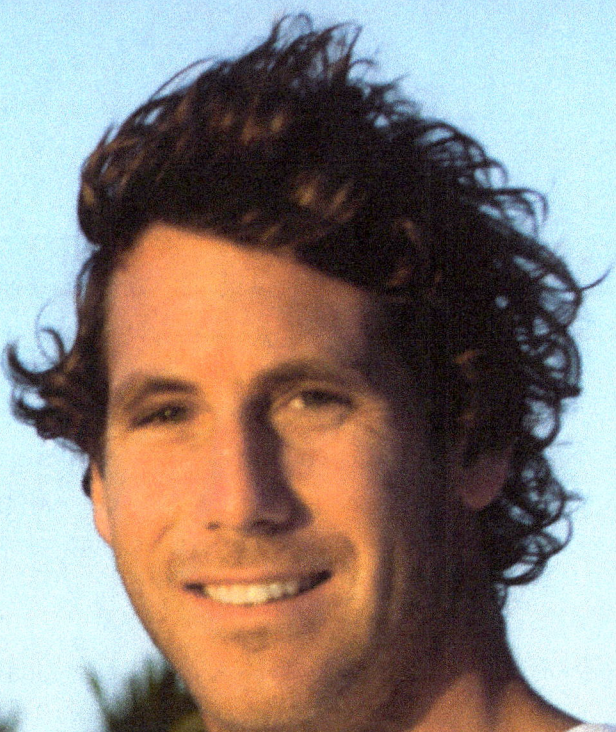

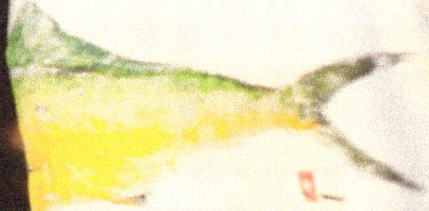

Creating your dream team

Now you are ready to voice your new goal – whether it is losing weight, running a half marathon, giving up smoking, going to the gym, taking up a new class or quitting sugar!

Once you bravely put this out there, you will notice that people might test your conviction, lead you astray, challenge the fact you can do it, or even overtly not support you at all. It can be really confronting for people to see you step up and put your goals into action, and it's human nature for people to raise opposition to others' goals, particularly when they wish they could get up and do something themselves.

You may find that the ones you love the most are the least supportive. Well, don't take this personally. As the saying goes, it tells you more about them than it does about you – so you need a fast and genuine strategy for support and encouragement, both at home and within your wider social circle.

Despite the challenges you may face, do not give up and don't get discouraged! This is an important lesson to engage in your own journey, your own goals and take control for yourself.

Your dream team is comprised of people who are truly:

*   ★ **Authentic:** they practice what they preach and are happy for your successes, too.
*   ★ **Knowledgeable:** especially if they are in a coaching or trainer role for you.
*   ★ **Positive:** about themselves, the world and you as well.
*   ★ **Genuinely interested:** in you and your achievements, milestones, trials and tribulations.

Finding your dream team

One of the top 5 tasks I give my clients, wherever they are based in the world, is to find their dream team. What on earth does this mean?

Simply put, it means that once you embark on your journey towards becoming your personal best, it s crucial to have the right people around you to encourage, support and be excited for you as you go through each milestone.

Your dream team can be made up of family, friends, a mentor, your trainer, coaches, your work colleagues, people you workout with, a wellness community online or those you get advice from.

Whoever they are, they must genuinely want to see you succeed. Your dream team can even include your kids as you engage them in your goals and show them how much their support means to you.

If you are hiring a personal trainer they MUST be vested in your success, tailoring your program and supporting you along the way. This is not about how good they look; keep in mind that you are set to become a reflection of their knowledge, professionalism and what they do, so make sure you're working with the best of the best!

Surrounding yourself with others who share a similar journey, outlook and approach can make the world of difference. There are some wonderful trainers, studios and gyms that are such a good fit, they form an 'extended family'. Consider joining into local group fitness sessions, as you may meet some fantastic training buddies along the way.

You will discover a whole new world, and potentially an inspiring and like-minded set of friends and mentors, who want to see you succeed.

As you venture into a new, healthier lifestyle **there may be some 'support casualties** along the way. There will be some friends, family members or colleagues who are not a part of your clean, healthy-living mentality. Keep focused on what is important to you and the long-term benefits of wellness and vitality, versus the short-term gratification of fitting in.

Asking for support

I truly believe that one of the main things that can let us all down in life is the inability to ask for help. Regardless of what your goal is, if you have the courage to simply ask for support – at work, from friends, from your family – you have a much greater chance of successfully reaching your goals.

Getting those you love on board:

★ **Communicate your goals** and be clear about how important this is for you.
★ **Empower your family** by asking them for their love, help and support.
★ **Make a fun schedule** that you can put on the fridge for your kids to give YOU gold stars when you achieve your nutrition and fitness goals each day.
★ **Include them** in your fitness and healthy eating journey. Cook together, go outside and be active together on weekends or in the afternoon, or discover a new sport you can do as a family, like biking, stand up paddling or just long walks with the dog.

★ **Lead by example.** If you're making positive, healthy changes, rest assured you are setting a great example for your children on how to look after their health and wellbeing.

What about support at work and play?

★ **Only share** your goals with those you care about and trust – this is your personal space and it's no place for dream stealers.

★ **Be polite,** but firm. If and when people try to tempt you away from your goals with 'just one drink' or 'just one cupcake', remind them politely and don't give in to temptation out of a desire to not rock the boat.

★ **Organise a fun run** or group activity within your workplace that creates a sense of team spirit around you.

★ **Book time out** in your diary for your own wellbeing – whether it's taking a proper lunch break with a colleague, enjoying some fresh air during a walk or buddying up with a friend for spin class or Zumba after work. Create time and accountability and follow up with actions, not words.

★ **Connect to a community** online. It might be a Facebook community or an online forum; I also offer a free VIPFIT membership where you can receive motivational tips and tools via email each week. Start right now by connecting with Team Vitality at Facebook.com/VitalityTheBook.

Goal Setting: Managing Milestones

Managing milestones is one of the most rewarding aspects of your new approach to health and fitness. While you want the habits and routines you create to ultimately become your new lifestyle, it takes some effort in the beginning stages to get there – and the motivational power of milestones can be an effective tool along the way.

I want to provide you with a clearer idea of how you can nourish your soul and your body, without having to turn your life upside down in the process.

My philosophy is all about integrating small, achievable health and wellbeing habits into your daily life. You can achieve this by:

- ★ Adding brief yet quality moments of exercise to your day – start with the 10-minute or 10-rep rule.
- ★ Stretching and focusing on breathing and appreciating the moment, giving you a healthy glow from the inside out.
- ★ Knowing which meals to chose and which ones to avoid when preparing meals for the family, eating out with clients, travelling or sitting in the office.
- ★ Working out ways to decrease internal stress effects on your body and promote a lean body, without silly diets.
- ★ Being kind to yourself and bringing balance into your well-planned week.
- ★ Ensuring you have the right balance of nutrients, protein, carbohydrates and natural fats that your body needs to function at its best – I'll help you learn all of this as we go!
- ★ Balancing your hormones by looking at nutrition for the energy/blood sugar balance and the nutrients you need to workout and keep things ticking along.

If you follow the plan and are inspired to look for healthy alternatives, to be prepared and to take responsibility for your personal best, then the sky truly is the limit!

- ★ Purpose with food – it's about knowing what to eat and how to eat, so that you start to feel in control. Add some new meals and menu options that you can cook at home that your kids/friends/partner will also enjoy.
- ★ Decreased body fat/measurements from your hard work and determination from the day you start. Use a tape measure and jump on the scales – once a week, not every day.
- ★ Increased energy levels - feeling more sustainable energy, better sleep, vitality.
- ★ Renewed confidence – with something to aim for, you'll experience renewed confidence as you achieve new personal goals – because you KNOW you can do it!

In the first four weeks, here s what you should expect to feel and see from your hard work and determination:

PHASE	WEEK	GOAL	PREPARATION	DISCIPLINE	RESULTS
1	1-2	Full Throttle	Max	No excuses	Energy to train – feel posture change, toning starts. New meals.
2	2-3	Consistency	Max – Moderate	Stick to the plan	Toned Abs & Fitness
3	4-5	Diversify	Moderate – Max	New dimension	Personal Challenge
4	Ongoing	Habit	Low – Natural	It's part of my life	Easy to maintain – others ask, "How do you do it?"

Preparation is the key to success and once you've mastered that, it should all become a habit. You l also learn how to:

- ★ Enjoy adding small quality moments of exercises to your day
- ★ Stop later afternoon hunger snacks/large portions at home
- ★ Know what meals to chose when out with clients and traveling
- ★ Have regular and small portions throughout the day
- ★ Ensure you have the right balance of nutrients, protein, carbohydrates and natural fats that your body needs to function at its best.

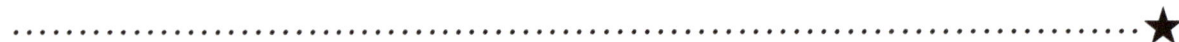

....★

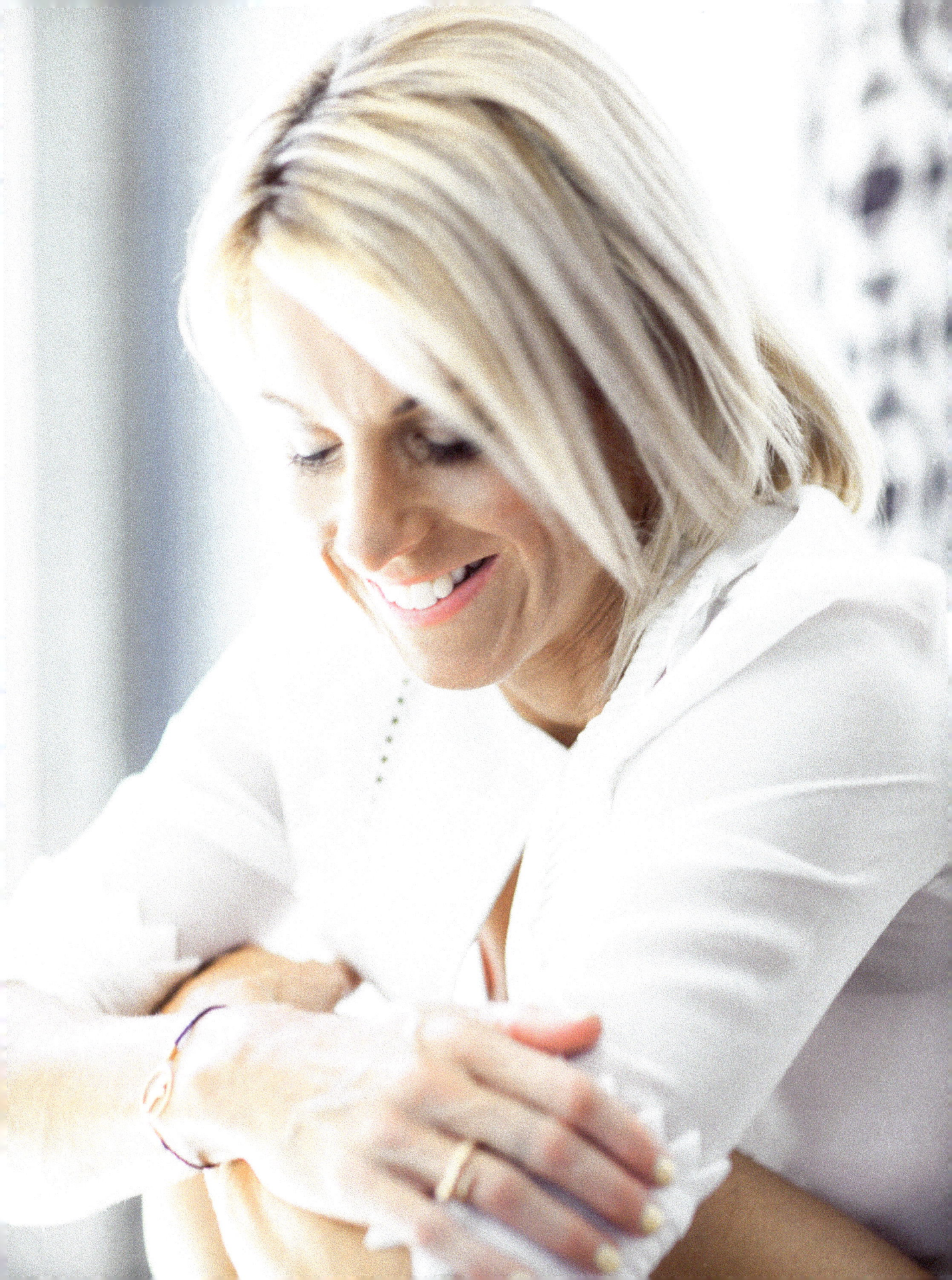

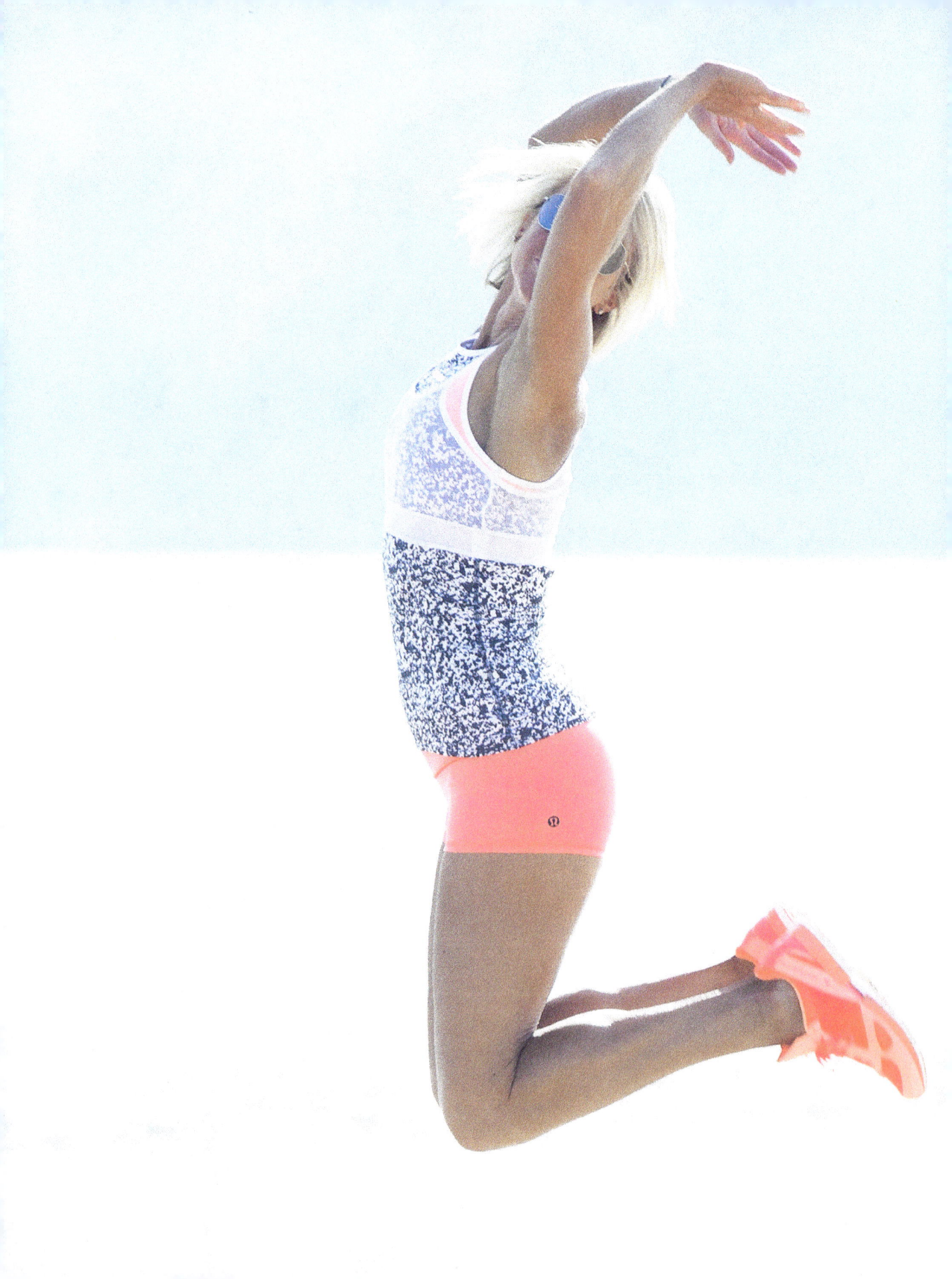

CHAPTER TWO: FRESH AIR

The concepts of exercise, fitness and working out can be overwhelming if you have been out of action for a while or if you're just not feeling the mojo.

But there's no time like the present to start making healthier, more active choices. Remember, even the pros had to start somewhere and I can guarantee you that everyone around you exercising will be focused on their own goals, rather than noticing what you are doing.

They key to success? Don't leave your health and fitness as the last priority on your agenda each week. Book it in as your first and least-negotiable appointments, and then head outside and enjoy your active lifestyle, without fear of what you may look like or what level you are at.

And remember: "Someday" is not a day in the week – only Monday to Sunday are. And what an opportunity we have to use them!

3 tips to put fitness first

1. Get Outside!

Really: lace up those shoes and make a promise to yourself that you will get out the door and start walking for 15 minutes without turning back. That s all it takes to get started. You don't have to commit to an hour of strenuous activity or an activity you "don't have time for". You just have to get outside and move, and clear your head with some good old-fashioned fresh air.

So step outside, talk a walk in the morning or during your break and exercise as much as you can outdoors. Being in nature has an incredible way of allowing you to calibrate and put things into perspective. We are often our most creative when we reduce the clutter around us and free up mental space to allow fresh thoughts and ideas.

Psst: To stop making excuses about "not having enough time" to exercise and get out of the habit of thinking that fitness is about things you don't like doing. Instead, focus on the "get out the door" philosophy. If you just make that your mission, you ll never look back.

2. Change your mindset

You need to truly believe that fitness is important. If you are having fun browsing Pinterest, Instagram and Facebook for all the "fitspo" images, thinking, "Wow, I wish I could do that… look ike that… be that"… Then stop and ask yourself: do you really BELIEVE you can be fit, healthy and happy?

All the positive affirmations in the world are not going to help unless you work on your self-belief and authentically want to be the best version of yourself. You can change negative self-image with time, habit and most importantly **actions** that signal to your brain and body that you actually are committed to feeling great.

Talking and thinking about it are a start – actually doing it creates change".

3. Do what you love

Exercise, healthy food and fitness should be FUN. Don't think of it as working out or something you have to do, but rather, think about activities that make you say, "I want to do that!" Have fun while exercising and your overall fitness will improve without you knowing it.

There are so many active elements in our lives, hopefully you can find at least one or two that make you feel fantastic as you do them. Try:

Running, Walking, Cycle, Swim, Group Classes at the Gym, Ballet, Barre, Pilates, Outdoor Fitness, Bootcamp, Football, Volleyball, Yoga, Skipping, Skiing, Mountain Biking, Surfing, Kite Surfing Stand Up Paddle, Down Wind Paddle Paces, Tennis, Golf, Trail Running – the list is ENDLESS!

Fit tip:
Limited to the gym for your workout, due to where you live or work? Look for a space that is fresh, clean, inspiring inside and promotes balance – rather than a 'manufactured', impersonal gym environment with heaps of overhead lighting and rows and rows of equipment.

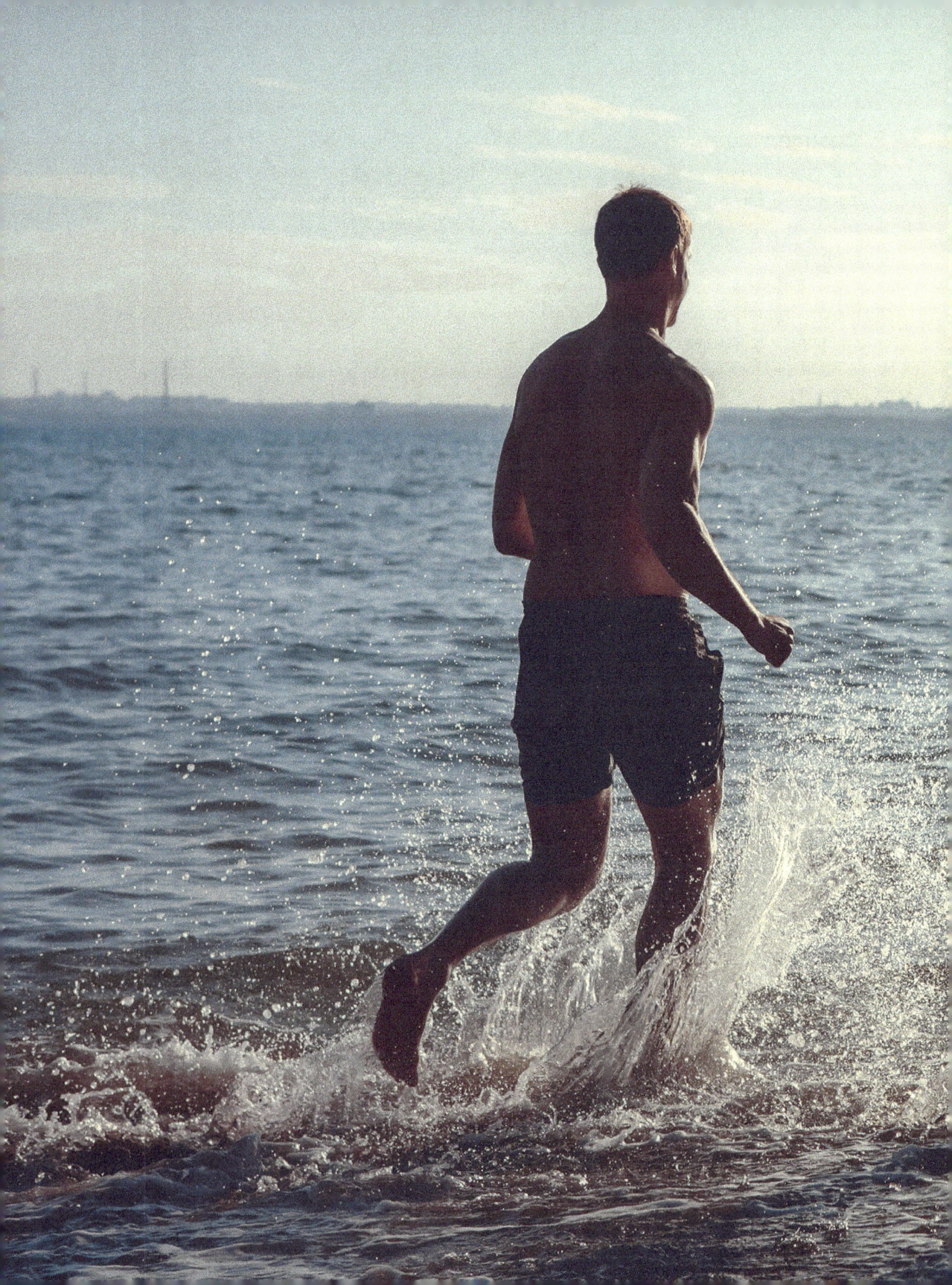

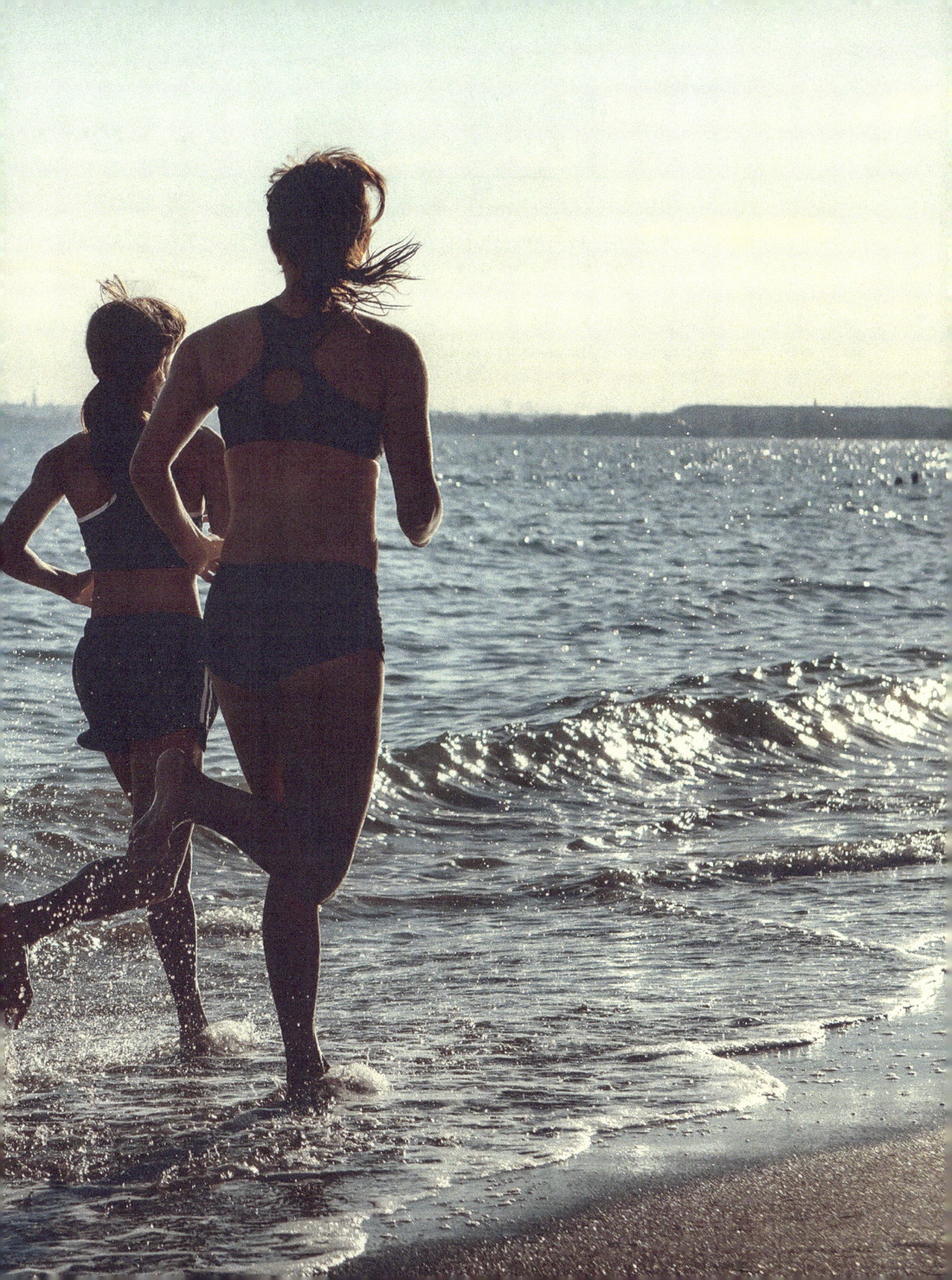

Nature is your gym

The more you tune in with your body and start to remember the elements of functional fitness, the more you can make life your gym. Working out does not have to be confined to a gym or with certain equipment. Nature can be an inspiring training partner and backdrop to reaching your fitness potential.

Once you start using nature as your gym, it s pretty hard to stop. I firmly believe our environment inspires us and that in order to find balance, a sense of peace and switch off from the world, nothing beats a wonderful spot in nature. That s why nature makes a great gym.

Even if it s just a few minutes a day that you get to top up on some fresh air, it can help to create an entirely different experience and mindset. We need to step away from computer screens, overhead lights, neon signs and mobile phones just for a moment to engage in the world around us. It is truly calibrating!

"Whether you're an ocean lover or are drawn to the mountains and snow, there are ample possibilities to workout, without even realising it."

5 KEY BENEFITS OF A HEALTHY BODY
 ★   Heart health
 ★   Injury prevention
 ★   Peak mental performance
 ★   Prevention of illness
 ★   Cellular health

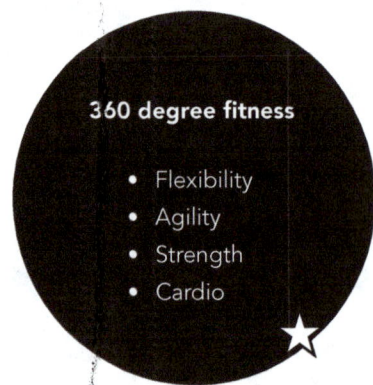

360 degree fitness

- Flexibility
- Agility
- Strength
- Cardio

The Wake up Workout™

Reality check: most of us have trouble being motivated and keeping workouts consistent. If this sounds like you, I recommend you wake up and work out straight away. By getting your exercise in before daily tasks and a busy life intervenes, you are less likely to put off your workout until the next day.

What's more, it kick starts your metabolism by increasing your body temperature after sleeping, and gets fresh blood fl owing around your body, which helps with a healthy heart and mind.

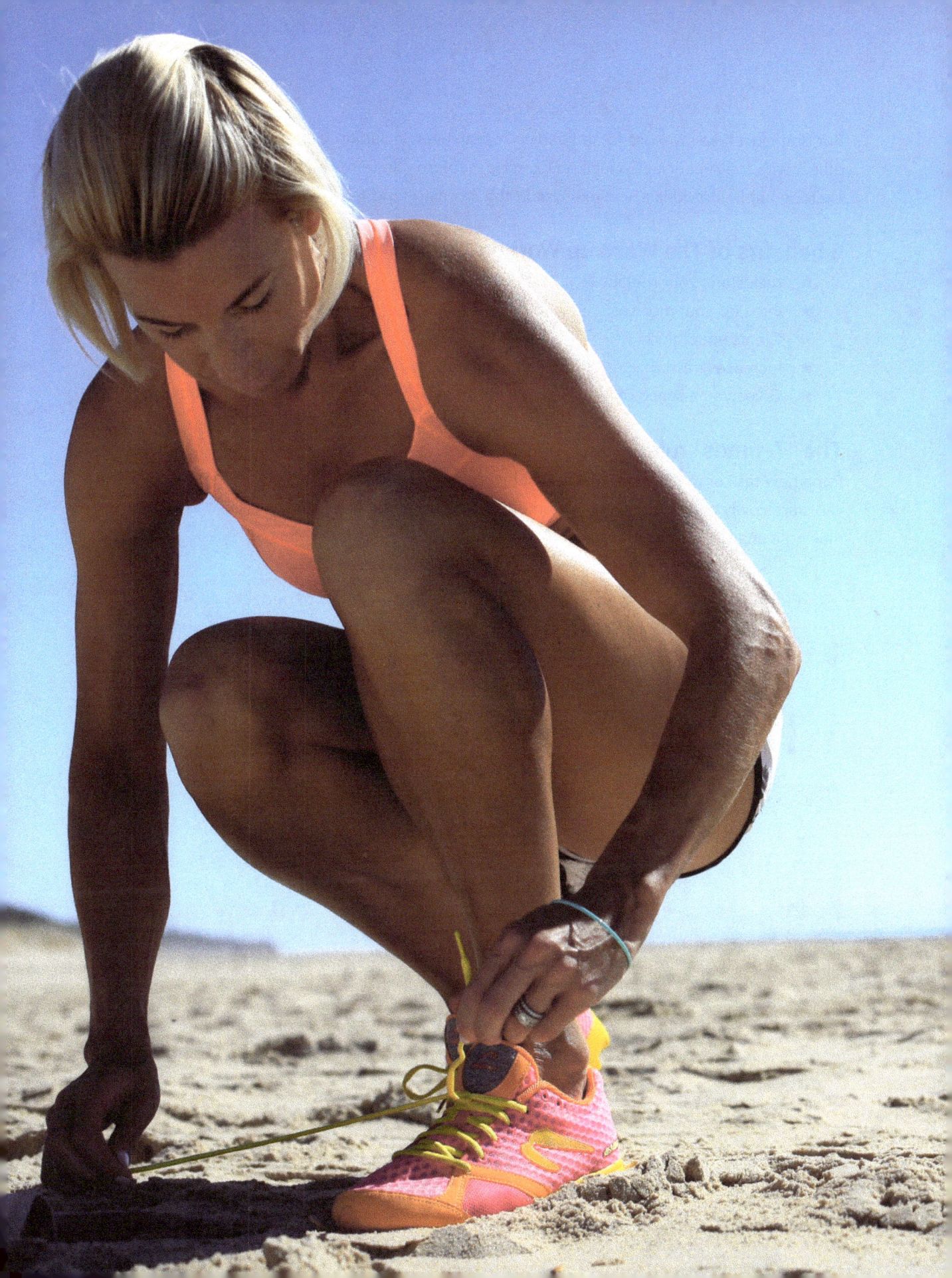

But don't just take my word for it. Leading researchers, including Cedric Bryant, PhD, chief science officer with the American Council on Exercise, confirm: "In terms of performing a consistent exercise habit, individuals who exercise in the morning tend to do better."

5 benefits of The Wake up Workout™:
★ Kick starts your metabolism
★ Fires up your muscles
★ Clears your mind
★ Increases fresh oxygen for a healthy heart
★ Gives you a sense of accomplishment after completing your workout for the day

The "7-times" rule
For a new task or routine to become a habit, we must set the goal for seven times in a row. You can start slowly or kick into high gear immediately, depending on your goals and enthusiasm for making a change! Aim to do this for 7 consecutive days:

SUPER EASY START:	As soon as you wake up get straight out of bed. DO NOT hit the snooze button. If your snooze button happens to have arms and legs, set an alarm for 10 minutes before your children normally wake up. Do 10 push-ups, 10 crunches and 10 deep breaths in and out. That's it.
EASY START:	As soon as you wake up get straight out of bed. DO NOT hit the snooze button. Do the Wake Up Workout.
ON A MISSION:	As soon as you wake up get straight out of bed. DO NOT hit the snooze button. Throw on your work out gear, grab your iPod loaded with your fave music, head out the door and run or walk, even cycle, for 15 minutes one way – turn round and come back. Job DONE. Double the time if you have it.

EXERCISE 1: THE PLANK

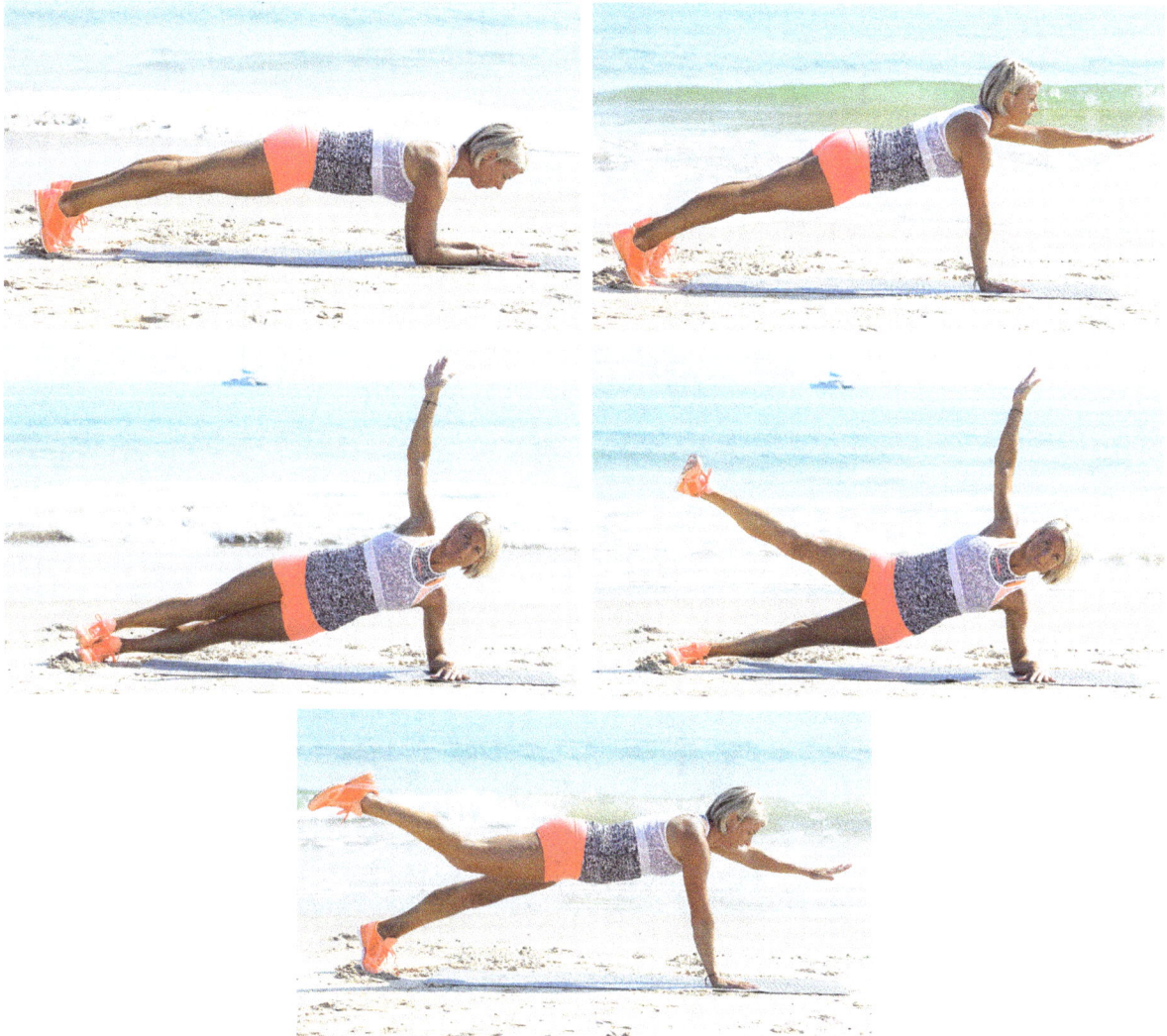

★ Rest on your forearms with your body in one line from head to hip to heel.

★ Tighten abs and lift onto your toes.

★ Push through to your toes, engaging your core and all muscles from top to toe.

★ Keep your hips in line with your shoulders.

★ Remember: technique is more important than time. Keep your eyes 'soft' and focus on your breathing.

★ Start with 5-10 seconds and build up to 60 seconds. Repeat if time permits.

EXERCISE 2: THE CLASSIC CRUNCH

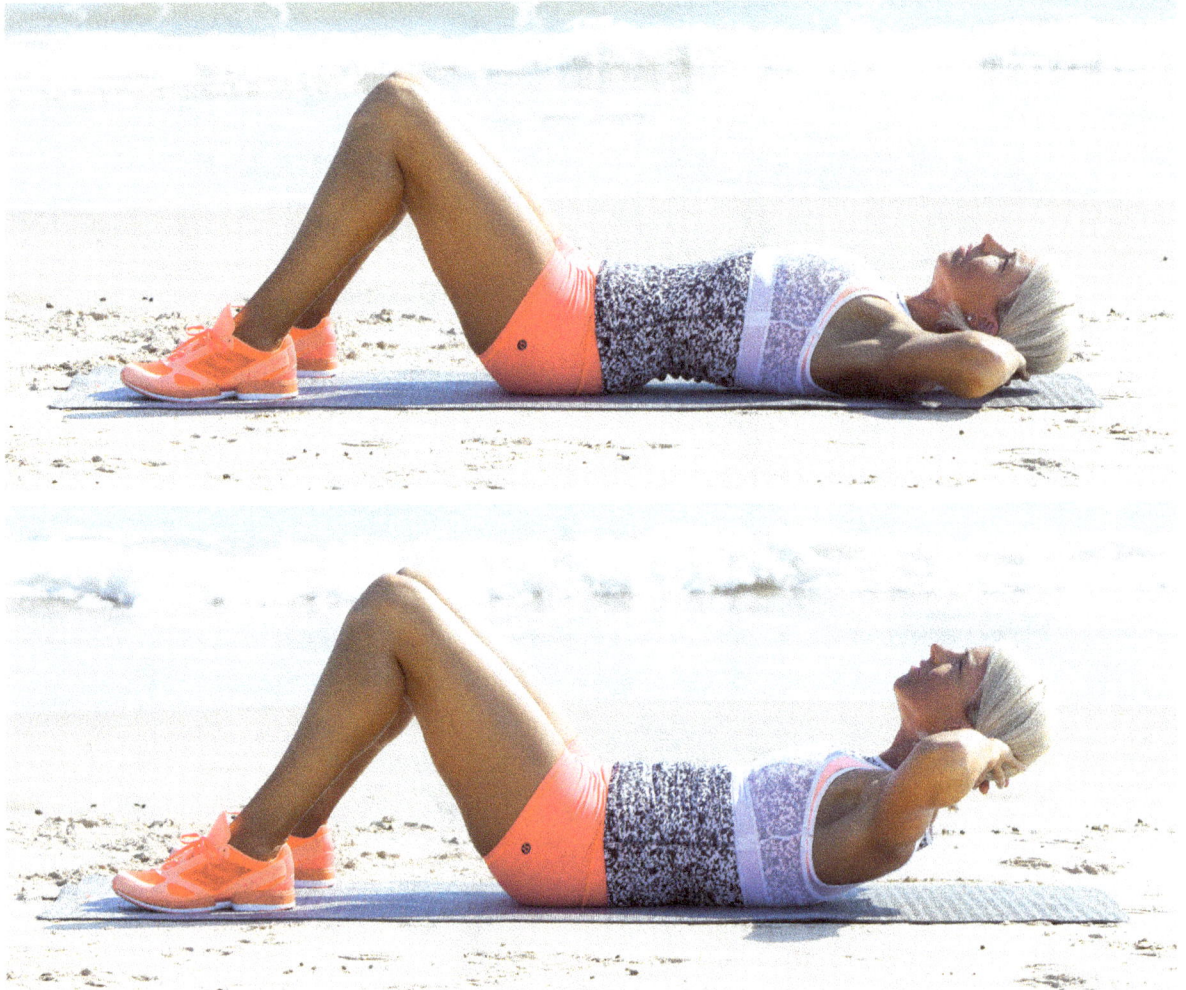

★ Start position is with your shoulders and head slightly raised.

★ Lie so the middle of your back is firmly on the ground – push your belly button towards your spine.

★ Put your hands behind your head but keep your elbows back at all times – this is really important!

★ Imagine balancing a plate on your forehead. Pulse up towards the ceiling/sky, looking up all the time.

★ Raise your upper body off the ground in small controlled movements; keep this tension until you reach 15 to 30 reps, then come down completely to rest.

★ Repeat: 30 to 50 reps x 3 is ideal.

EXERCISE 3: THE PUSH UP

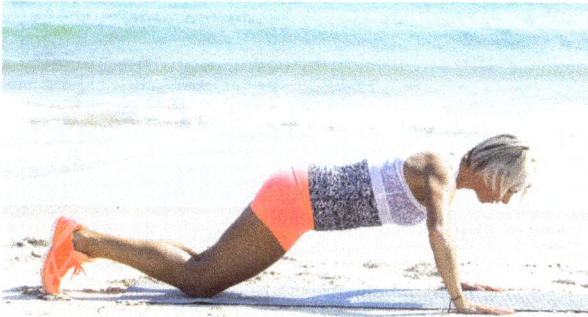

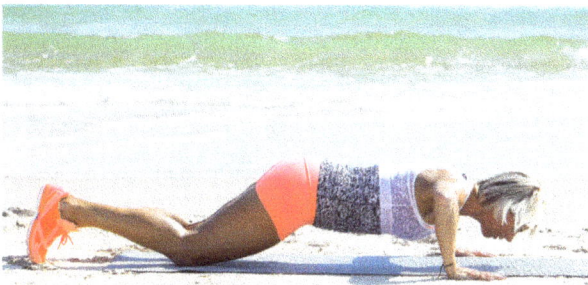

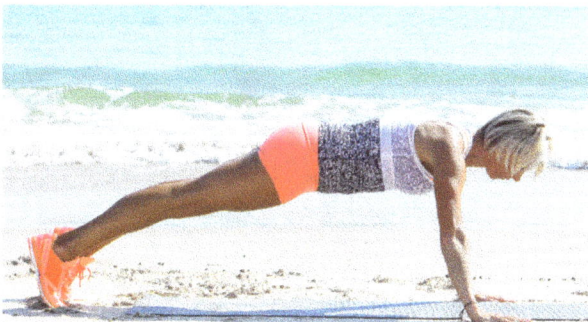

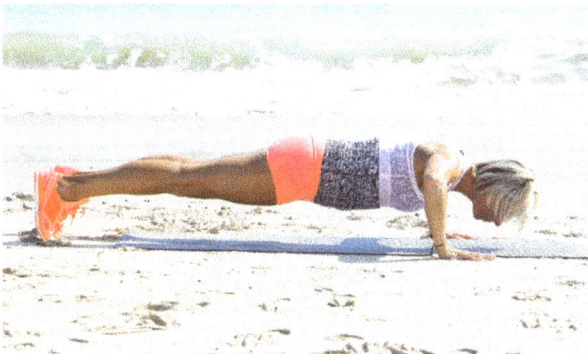

★ Keep your hands wide at all times and make sure your back is long with a full body extension. Even for the kneeling option, a long torso and wide hand position still applies.

★ Keeping your body in one line, head in line with your spine, take your feet to just within shoulder-width and hands wider than shoulder-width.

★ Complete full push up then back to start.

★ Hold abs tight and stable to prevent any strain in lower back.

★ Start with 5 and build up to 25 x 3 repeats.

EXERCISE 4: THE LOWER AB LIFT

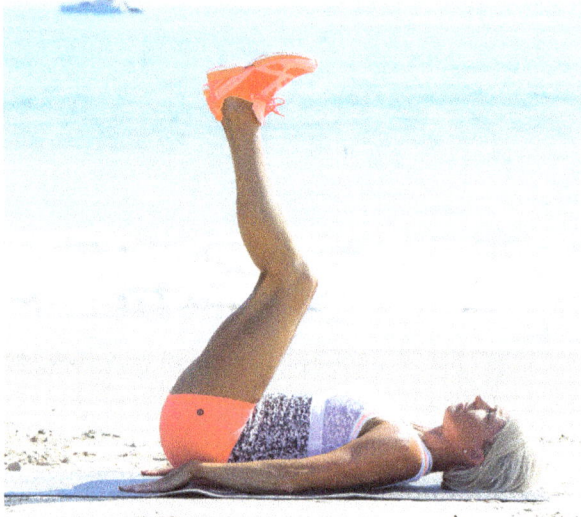

★ These are deceptively difficult! But the smaller the movement, the better results. Lie on your back, hands resting by your sides or behind your head.

★ Eyes to the ceiling/sky again.

★ With your hips and knees in line, extend legs to start position, feet flat to the sky, and toes flexed towards you.

★ Lift pelvis off the ground in small movements, hold slightly off the ground at the end of each rep: only come back down at the end of the set.

★ This is a good exercise to do with someone else to spot you to make sure your feet/legs stay as straight as possible and you push up to the sky rather than out.

★ Try 5 perfect ones and build to 25 x 3 repeats.

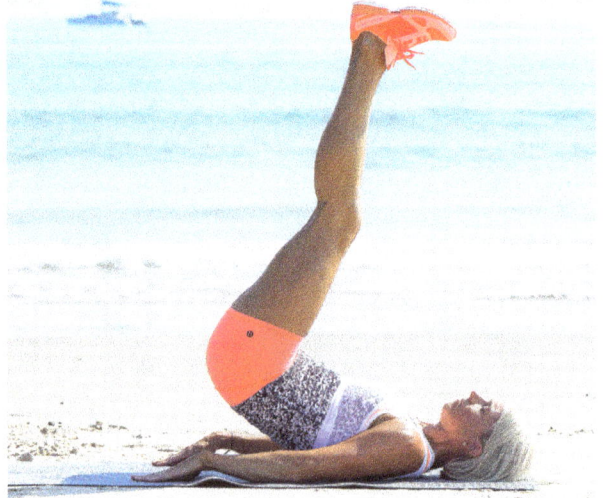

EXERCISE 5: THE CHILDS POSE

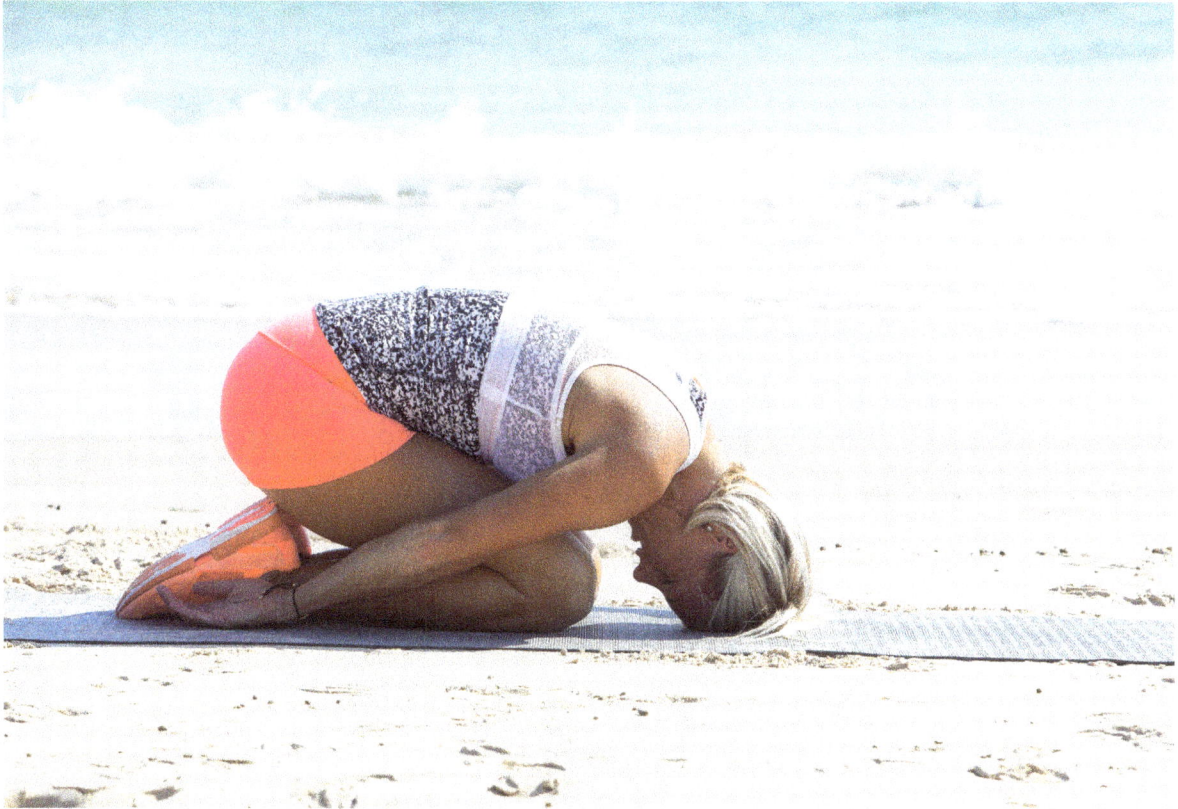

- ★ Roll gently onto your knees and hands.
- ★ Place forehead to the fl oor and gently place your hands by your sides palms facing up, or stretched out in front of you palms down.
- ★ Breathe in. Exhale slowly and deliberately.
- ★ Relax here for at least 10 counts of breath in and out.
- ★ Take your time to roll up from hips to shoulders.

That's it – you've completed the Wake Up Workout! This is a fail-safe, go-to exercise set for anywhere and anytime. I hope you incorporate this and other healthy-living moments into your day.

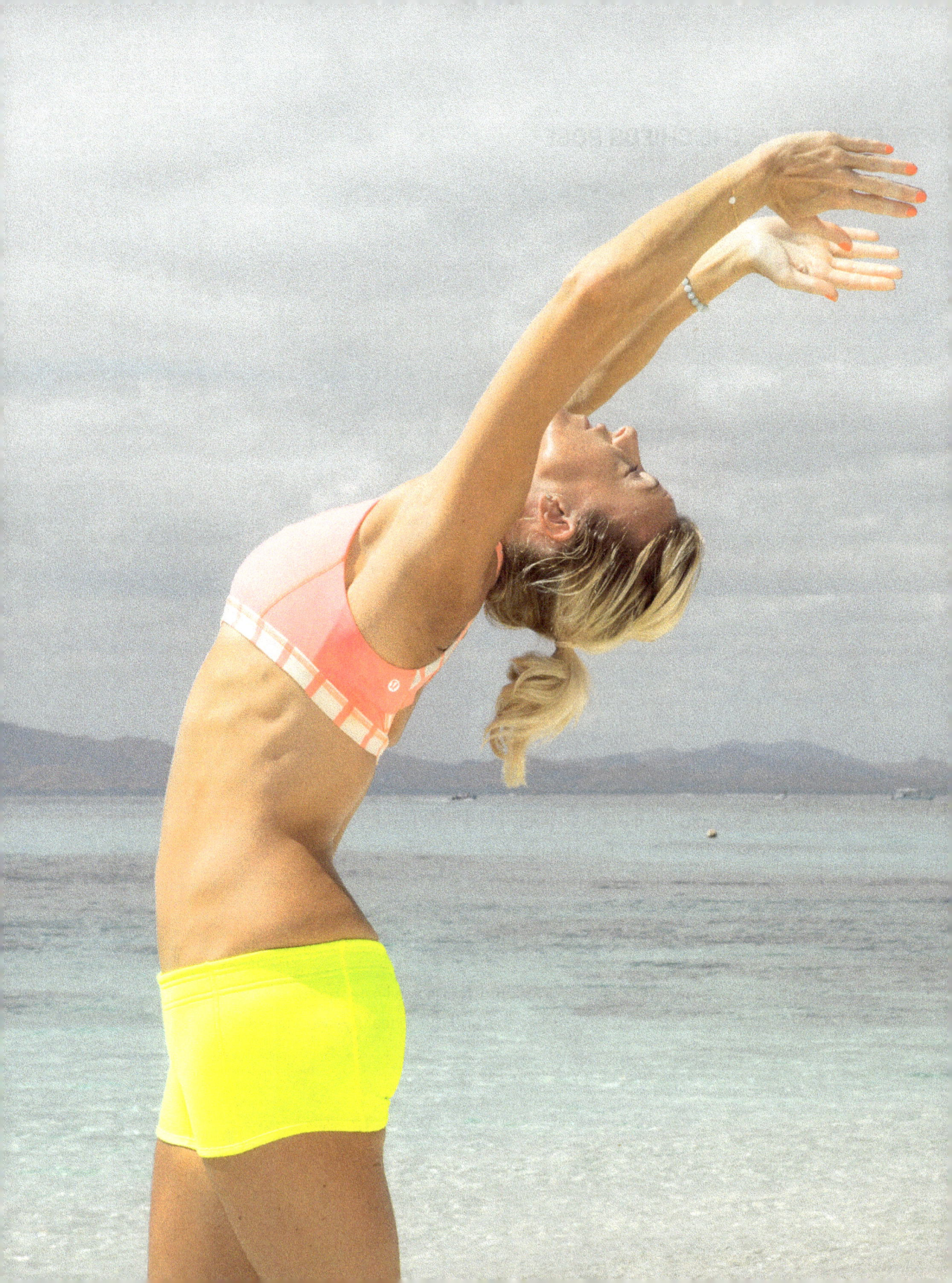

Yoga

Yoga is a wonderful body and mind workout that tones, strengthens the core, helps relax and improves flexibility. It is suitable for all levels of flexibility and fitness and can be completely adapted to work around injuries and even rehabilitate them.

Yoga strengthens and lengthens, providing work for your muscles to do but also helping to repair and regenerate on a cellular level. Flexibility is a crucial aspect to overall fitness. Weights, running, cycling and sitting all shorten muscles and tighten the body; stretching and yoga aid in injury prevention, circulation, decreasing levels of physical and mental stress and the effects these have on the body.

If you feel that you'd like to do yoga but you're intimidated by some of the moves you see posted on social media and Instagram, or perhaps think that it's about chanting and wheatgrass shots, let me assure you there are all types of yoga and differing levels of classes that may suit you and your needs.

Yoga is a journey; it's a personal one and not about comparing your milestones to anyone other than yourself. For 150% givers who have extremely busy lives, yoga and its practice can provide movements of calm in the storm.

My advice is to practice what you learn in the class or with your yoga instructor in between. Focus on one or two poses or breathing techniques that can form a part of your week. Even five minutes of concentrated breathing can clear your mind and help you connect with your intuition or balance out energy levels.

Nikki's fit tip:
Find a style of yoga that suits you.
There are so many available but not all
will serve your mindset or physical needs.
I love hot Power Yoga as it really is
a workout, not just a stretch.

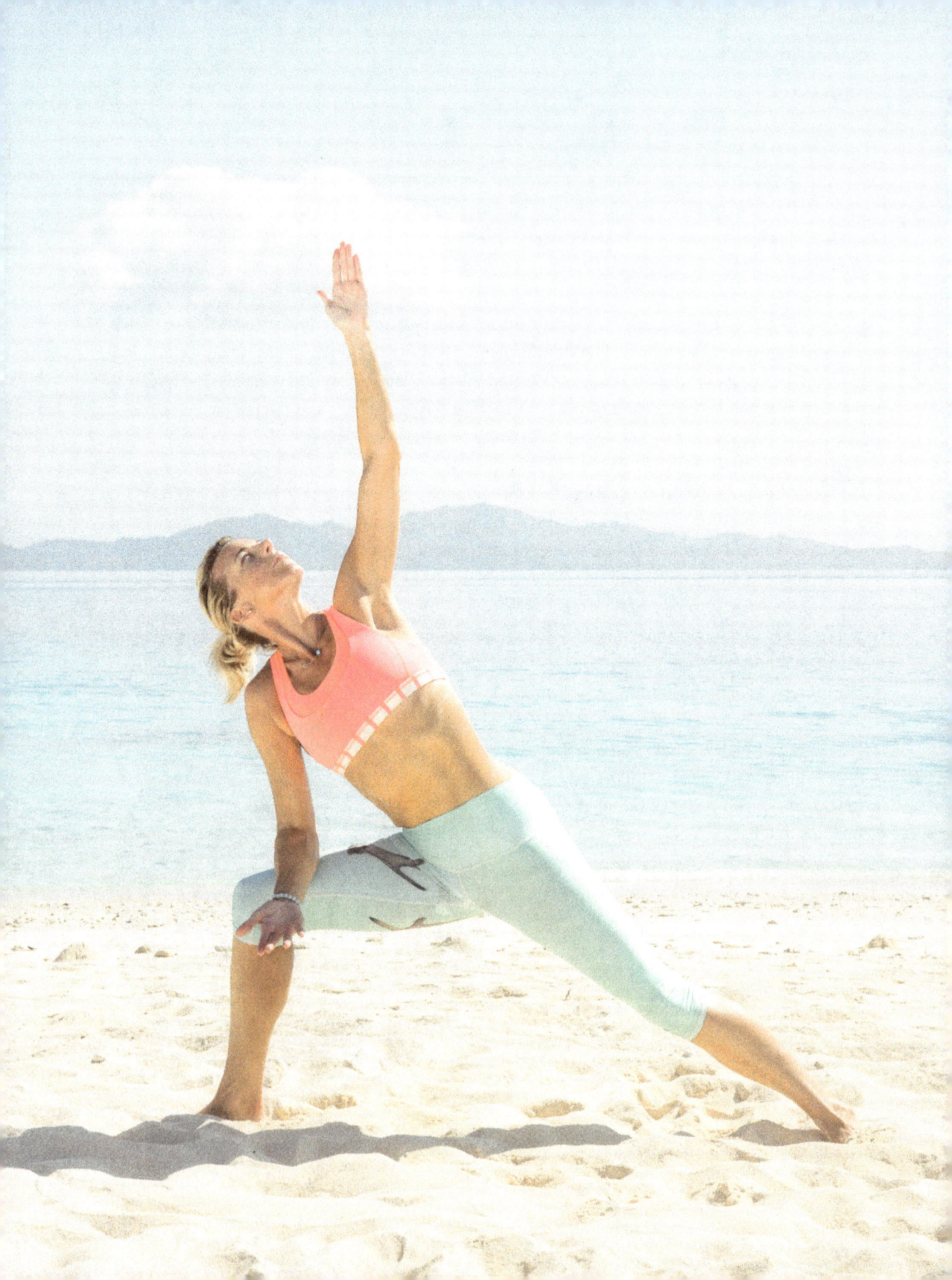

5 ways to incorporate it into your week:

★ Set aside time for a class each week

★ Research and practice 3 poses every day at home

★ Find out about mindfulness and focus on one mindful action or thought each day

★ Challenge yourself to a headstand competition with a friend or your kids (be careful and make sure you've got a buddy waiting to catch you if you fall)

★ Each day, think of something you're grateful for

For inspiration and step-by-step guides to more yoga poses, visit www.thevitalitycoach.com.au

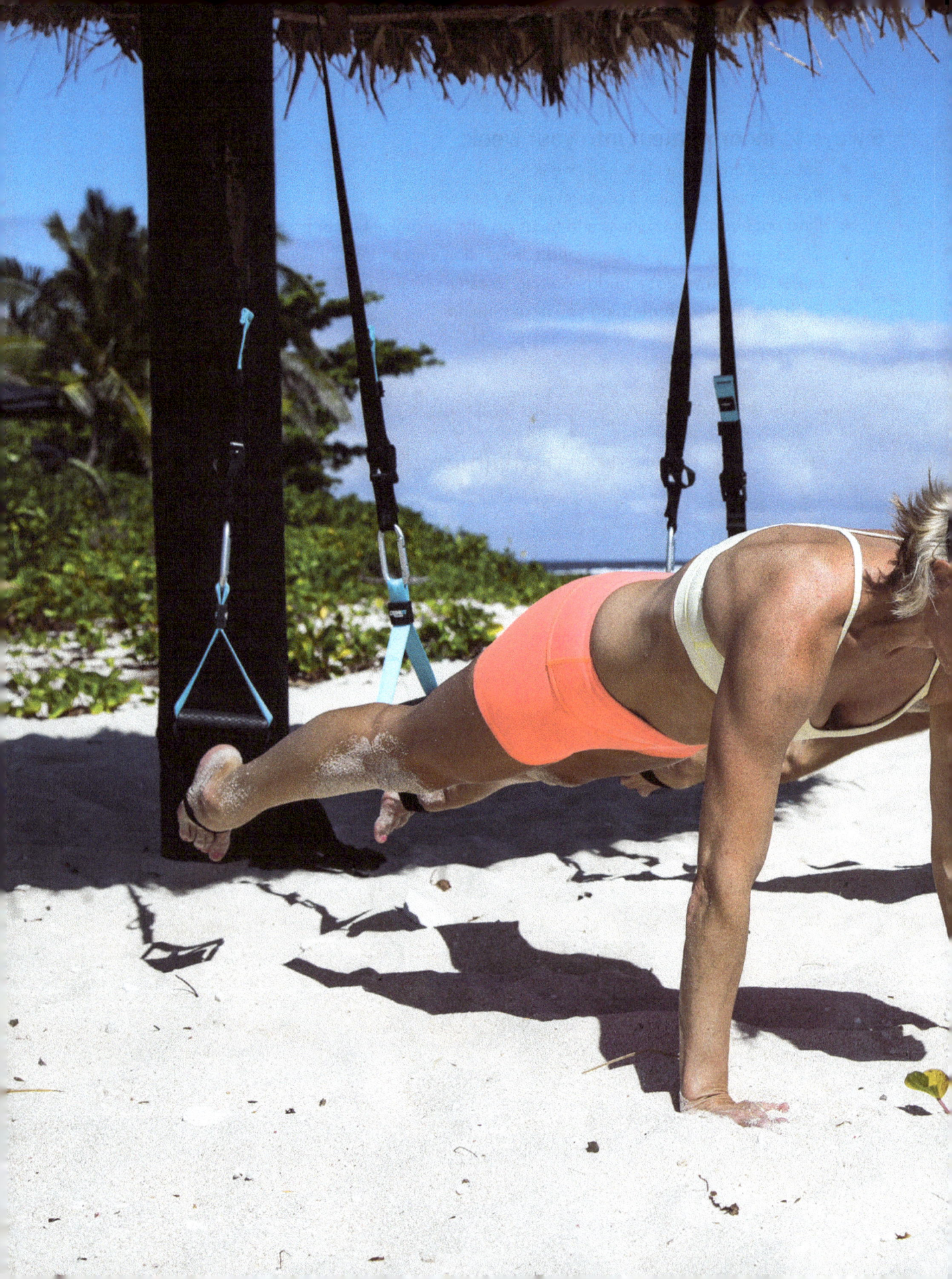

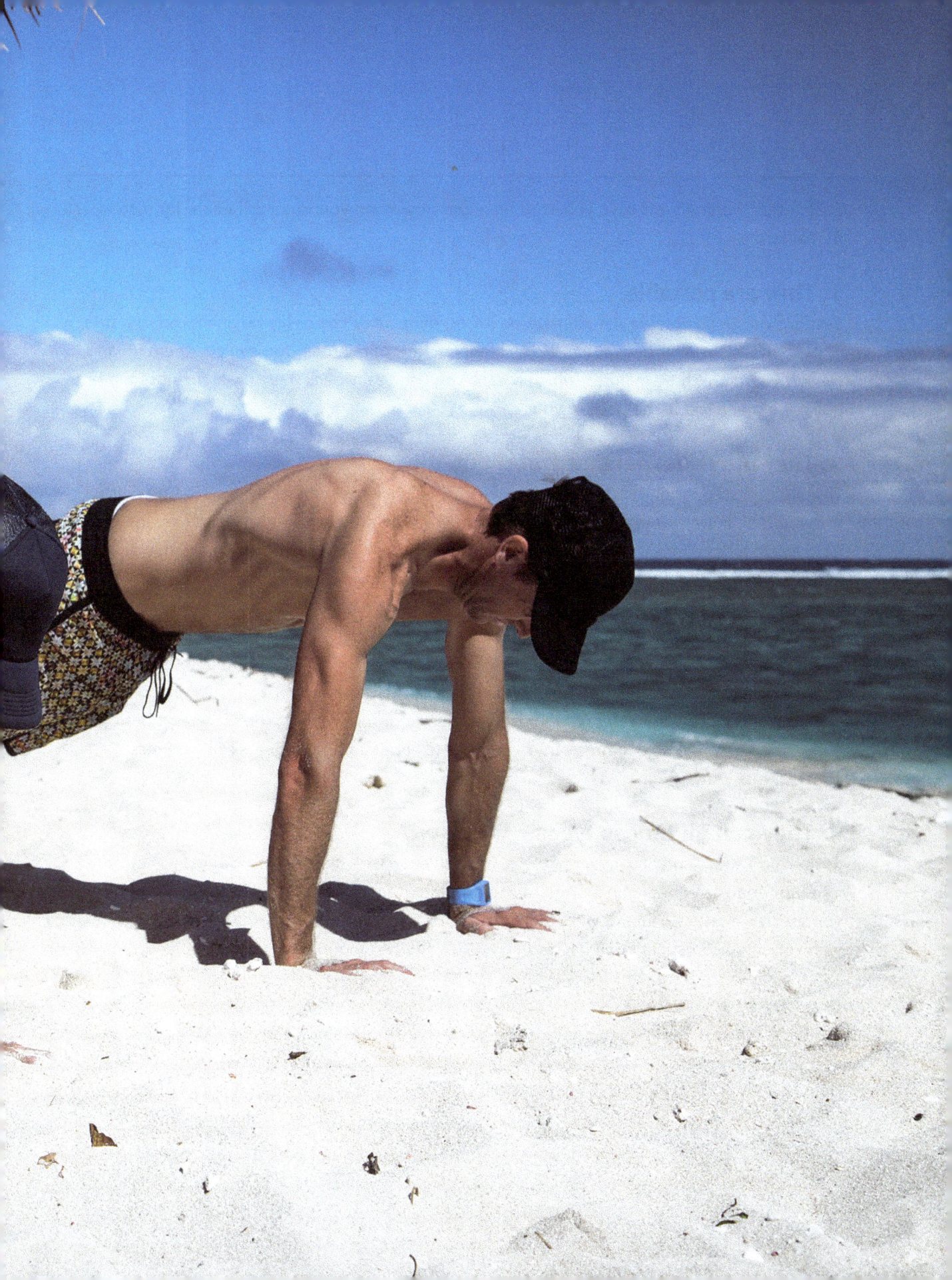

Suspension Training

Suspension workouts will save you both time and money on your road to health, for a number of reasons:

1. They are portable.

Suspension straps provide the ultimate travelling gym. They can easily be anchored to a tree, playground, door or strong structural beam in a matter of minutes. You can put them up and be ready to go in three minutes, which means you can easily pack them on a business trip, a holiday or even just in the back or your car.

2. They provide a balanced workout.

Training with suspension straps creates a necessary balance in your muscles, as it is very difficult to favour one muscle or the other during training. Because your body is the resistance, there is nowhere to hide. When you have the correct technique with suspension strap training, you know it, as you immediately go off-balance if you're not working the muscles equally on both sides.

3. They're effective.

Suspension training sessions can be super effective and quick; I love a 15-minute express session. You can use 1-2 minutes as interval training, then rest and repeat. Choose a body weight set to kick-start that works your bigger muscle groups to warm up, such as a basic squat, then go on to select three other exercises to super set, e.g. Squats | Chest Press | Triceps Press | Knee Tucks.

4. They suit all fitness types.

Suspension straps suit any level of fitness, as each exercise offers varying degrees of difficulty. The further away from the anchor point you are, the more difficult it is, as you have more of your body weight to contend with. Make sure as with any exercise/fitness element you check with your medical practitioner first and you follow the technique instructions.

5. They are low cost

For those who are budget-conscious, having your own "take anywhere gym" with a set of suspension straps is an ideal solution. An investment of $200 is all you'll pay for five years-plus of use.

3 exercises as a snapshot

1. Suspended Lunge – great for stability

Stand facing away from the the anchor point, place one foot in the straps and gently edge your other front foot forward. Ensure you have enough distance that your front knee is NOT over your toes when bent.

★ For stability keep your arms out in front of you. Lower your body by extending and bending the back leg and bending front knee to 90 degrees, into a lunge position. Keeping your front heel on the ground and ensure your back is long and straight. Core is engaged, eyes are forward and chin is not dropped towards your chest.

★ Balance your weight throughout your feet, not just the front foot but use the suspension of the back foot to evenly distribute weight.

★ Lunge down and return to a standing position. Repeat 10-15 times then change sides.

2. Chest Press

Facing away from the anchor point – take the handles in each hand and slowly lean out so that your arms are extended in front of you. Engage your core by pulling your belly button to your spine. Keep your eyes forward and chin up. Slowly bring your elbows back towards the anchor point – lowering your body into an incline chest press – then push out the arms to start position. Avoid dropping the hips and ensure your chest is upright. The CLOSER you are to the anchor point the more difficult this exercise is as it loads more body weight. Start further away to get the technique correct first. Don't pull on the straps it should be a smooth transition. Repeat this 10-15 times.

3. Suspended push up

One of my favourite exercise when I have limited time. Ensure the straps are fully lengthened to just a few inches off the ground. Kneel down and place your feet into the straps, then walk your walk forward on your hands.

Ensure your body is long and hips, heels and shoulders are all in line.

★ Keeping your back straight and eyes on the ground so your neck is in line. Extend arms into full push up position then come down by only bending your elbows to 90 degrees, with your nose towards the ground.

★ Repeat 10-15 times – or even just start with 5 perfect ones and build up from there.

★ For a more in-depth look at suspension training, visit www.TheVitalityCoach.com.au head to my YOUTUBE channel for all the videos www.youtube.com/VitalityCoachTV

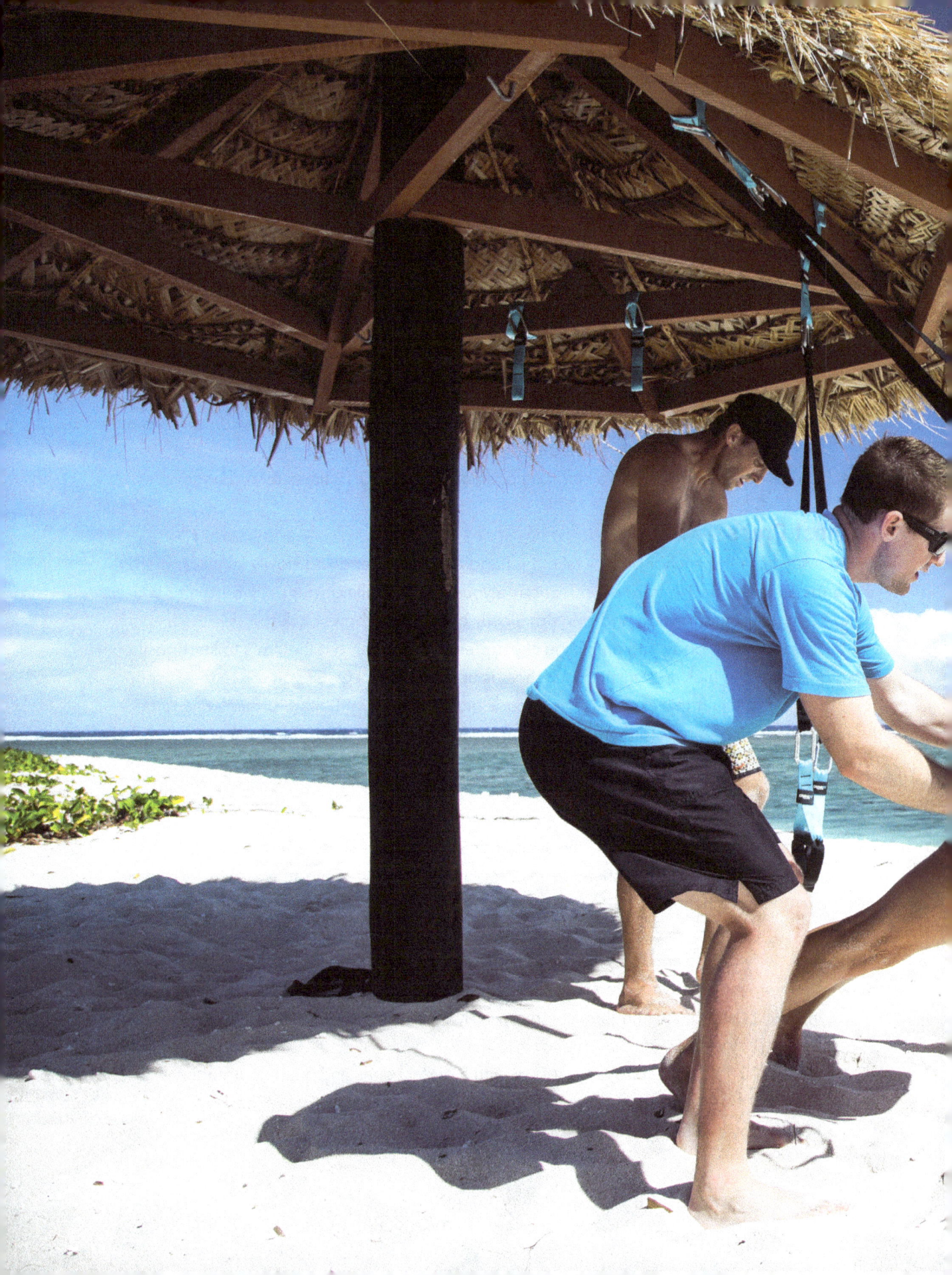

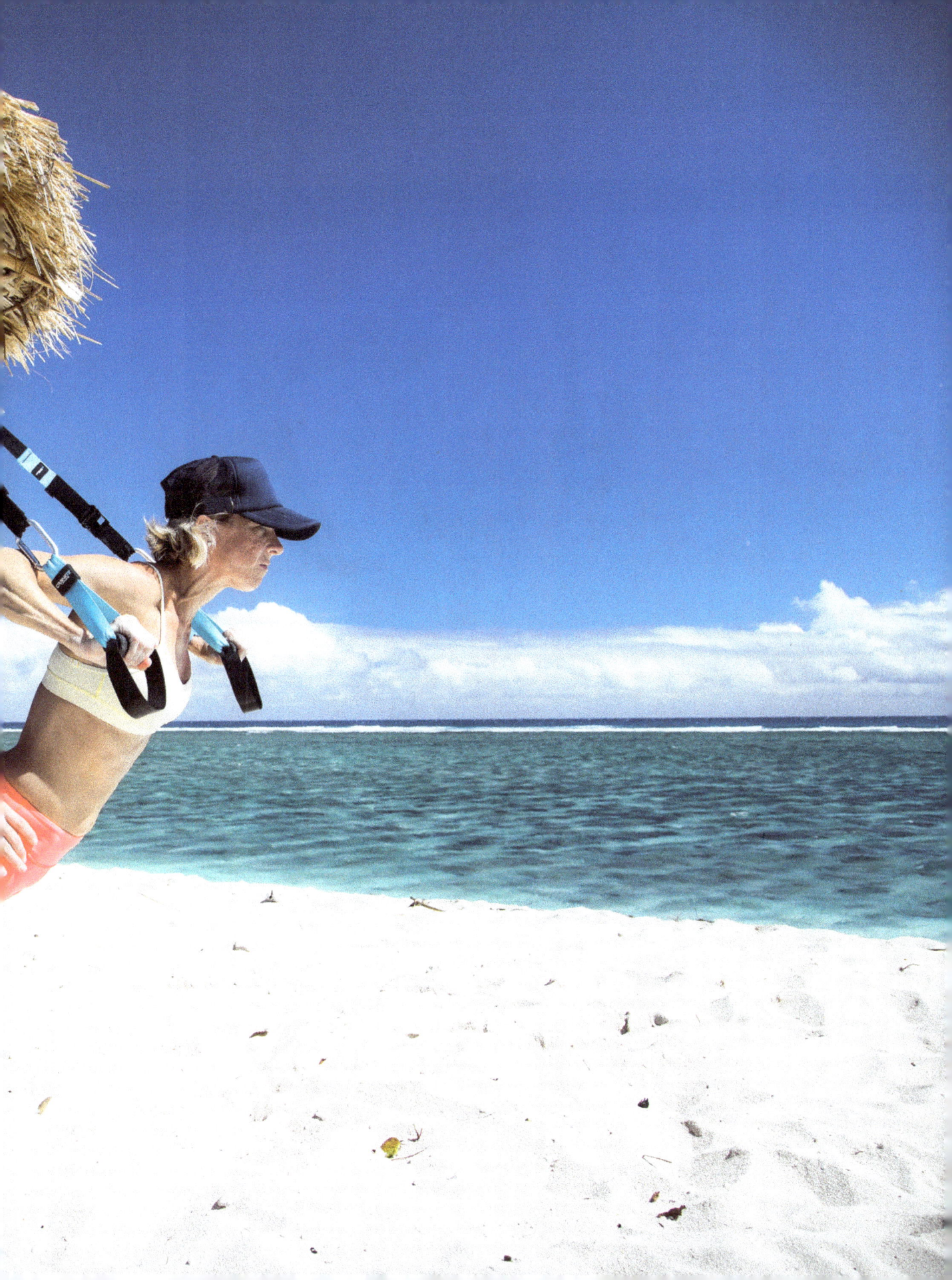

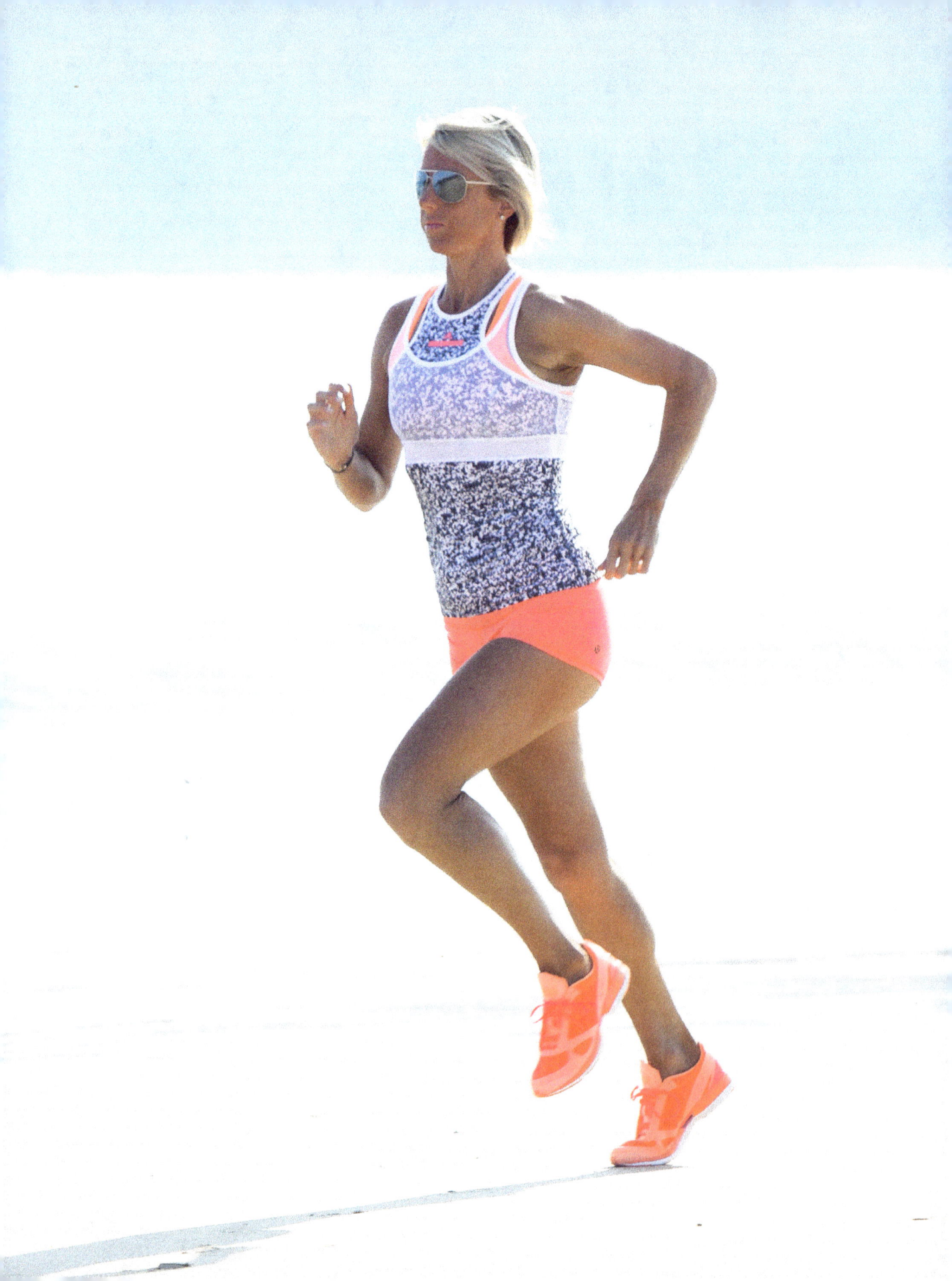

Running

Running for me is a complete body, mind and spirit workout. Whether it's 15 minutes of fresh air or just enough time to squeeze in a 5km run during a busy day, it helps me to calibrate, order my thoughts and blow out the cobwebs.

It offers a fantastic cardio workout, as well as being a great total-body toner. Increasing your blood flow and cardiac performance is wonderful for general health and wellbeing improving heart health and endurance.

There's a lot of hype around 'free running' shoes at the moment, which are designed to create a more natural running style by helping your toe land before your heel. If you've spent the last decade running in older-style shoes with your heel striking the ground first, this is going to be a big change for you. Don't underestimate the time it will take for your body to adapt. Go slow and be patient, or you'll risk injury.

My number 1 tip for beginners:
Make sure you have the correct running shoe and comfortable clothing that you can work out in. Speak to a specialist and test out a few pairs for comfort, being sure to select something that suits your foot, as well as the style and amount of running you plan on doing.

5 ways to incorporate running into your week:
- ★ Discover your local area on foot
- ★ Create your own running track and try to include some hills for extra intensity
- ★ Jog down to your local café and reward yourself with a coffee or fresh juice
- ★ Set a goal such as a fun-run, marathon or charity event for extra motivation
- ★ Get together with your friends on the weekend and go for a run before your lunch date

Inspired to get your run on? Visit www.TheVitalityCoach.com.au to download my ebook, *'RUN101: 4 Weeks To 5KM Ebook'.*

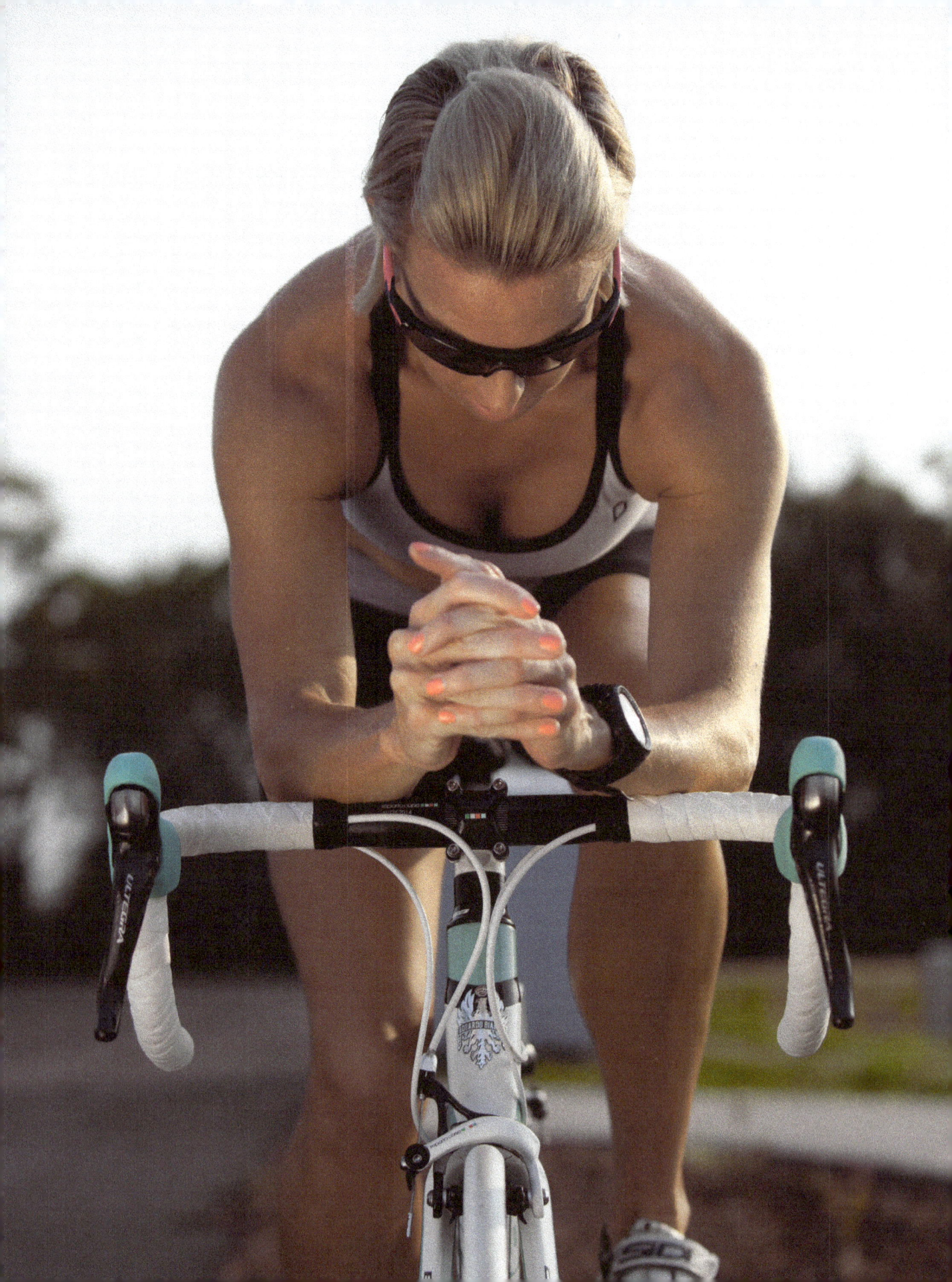

Cycling

What better way is there to take your fitness and super-toned body goals to the next level than by getting out on a bike?

Cycling is an ideal sport for everyday fitness warriors – all shapes, sizes, ages and fitness levels. It's never too late to get back in the saddle, or to learn! It can be liberating, it's social, effective for fitness and just fun discovering a new way to look at the city or area you live in.

It's also a sustainable form of fitness, both for your body and the environment; when you're working out like this you're not using electricity, air conditioning, or fitness machines. It's all pedal power.

Cycling worldwide has an incredible community feel, as it bridges the gap between ages, fitness levels and the sexes! It creates new friendships that might not have existed, brings people together in the face of adversity with charity rides and can provide a unique extended 'family' if you ride with a regular group.

So enjoy the ride – no matter what level of fitness this is one training platform that can fast track you in terms of fat loss, cardio fitness and strength!

Safety first!

Cars, trucks and buses make a bigger dent than a person on a bike; even if the vehicle is not moving, it's a hazard. Cycle with your head up and eyes forward at all times. Road cycling and even riding on paths needs some concentration as it's not just your actions, but those of other unpredictable elements that need your attention. While cycling is relaxing and fun, it's also crucial to know your safety 101.

Cycling is great for building your inner strength. Practice cycling with no hands (on the grass!) and notice how your stomach muscles engage.

5 ways to incorporate it into your week:
   ★ Ride all or part-way to work during the week
   ★ Cycle to your favourite coffee shop or the beach on weekends
   ★ Go mountain biking and explore your local forest
   ★ Join a cycle group
   ★ Set your sights on a competition in your area

Hooked on the idea of cycling? Head to www.TheVitalityCoach.com.au to download my ebook, 40 weeks to 40km'

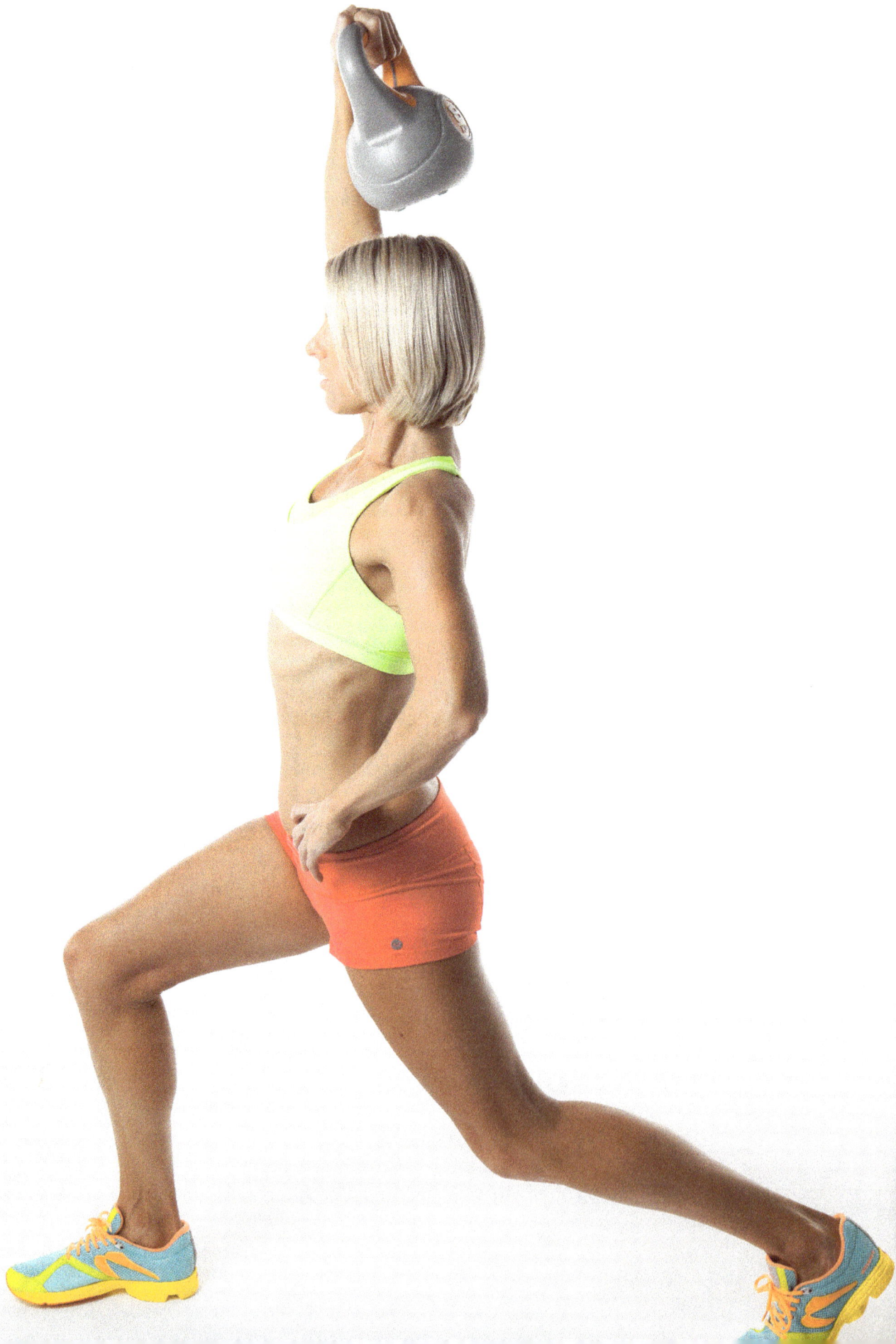

Kettlebells

These petite fitness accessories pack a powerful punch, as the dynamic movements not only target one area at a time, but also work out your whole body, as you need to balance and stabilise as you lift.

Moving the weight's centre of gravity outside of your palm means you need to use a range of muscles and directions of movement, recruiting other muscle groups.

Kettlebells are perfect for your at-home gym, as they take up a small amount of space and provide a fast, effective workout and a range of exercises that can be included in an existing regime.

They're ideal for those who want to increase their forearm strength and improve cardio fitness, as the exercises can be fast-paced and really get the heart rate up. Plus, the more muscles you use with each movement, means more time-efficient training.

Nikki's fit tip:
Kettlebell swings are fantastic exercises that work your muscles as they decelerate the weight and hold your body in balance. However, because of the inertia, they can be dangerous and many injuries occur with poor technique. As always, focus on technique before increasing weight and repetition.

Keep it simple, keep doing it, keep the results.
The better you look after your body, the better your body will look after you.

5 ways to incorporate it into your week:

★ Add a Kettlebell exercise to your morning regime
★ Try a class at the gym – I've even seen Kettlebell Yoga offered in some studios!
★ Keep your Kettlebell close to the TV and jump up to do 5 reps of a different exercise each ad break
★ Head outdoors and include your Kettlebell in a circuit
★ Meet up with a friend and show them how to use it (once you've mastered it yourself)

Beginners take note:

Ensure you choose a weight that is relevant to your level; avoid getting one too heavy as it will compromise your technique and in some cases you can injure yourself. Go slow and practice these exercise as an extension of other workouts.

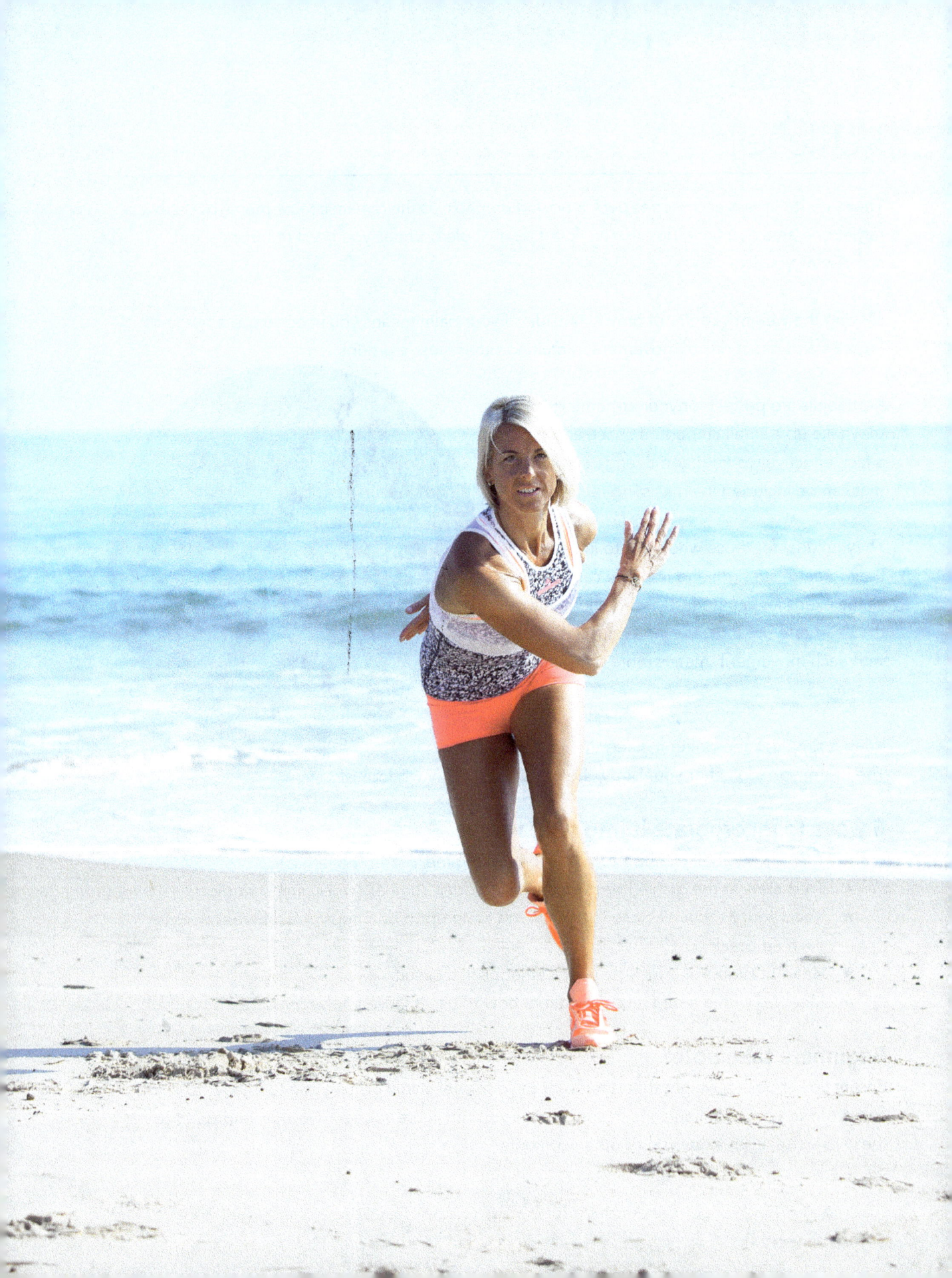

H.I.I.T. High Intensity Interval Training

High intensity training is so much fun, and best of all for busy people, it can be knocked out in less than half an hour!

H.I.I.T. is all about short, intense bursts of exercise that create incredibly powerful results.

Each session usually lasts for 20 minutes or less. The program kick-starts your metabolism and raises your heart rate above 75% to 90%, before resting for a minute or two, and then getting back into the zone again for another 2-3 minutes. Short bursts with regular rest and a short overall workout time makes it the ideal workout for busy people.

The post-workout metabolism boost that high intensity training provides is sometimes referred to as the after-burn.

Both cardio and strength routines can be high intensity, as long as they get your heart pumping over 75% and start working your heart on an anaerobic level. This type of training is ideal for body weight and exercise with weights as well.

Nikki's fit tip:
Form and technique are super important—don't sacrifice them for rushing through the time to increase reps.

Mini H.I.I.T. workout:

Kick start your cardio and interval training with this little mini workout, which utilises high-intensity body-weight exercises to get your heart rate up, burn calories, and supercharge your metabolism.

Exercise	Reps	Time	Active Rest Time
Squat with Jump	As many as you can	45 sec	15sec
Lunges	As many as you can	45 sec	15sec
Push Ups	As many as you can	45 sec	15sec
Bicycle Crunch	As many as you can	45 sec	15sec
REPEAT THIS SET 3-4 TIMES			

★ Add hand weights to lunges and squats as you build your strength.
★ Do these four moves back-to-back, completing as many reps as you can in the amount of time.
★ Rest for one to two minutes, then repeat.
★ Build up your time and reps each week by adding 10-15 seconds of time to each exercise.

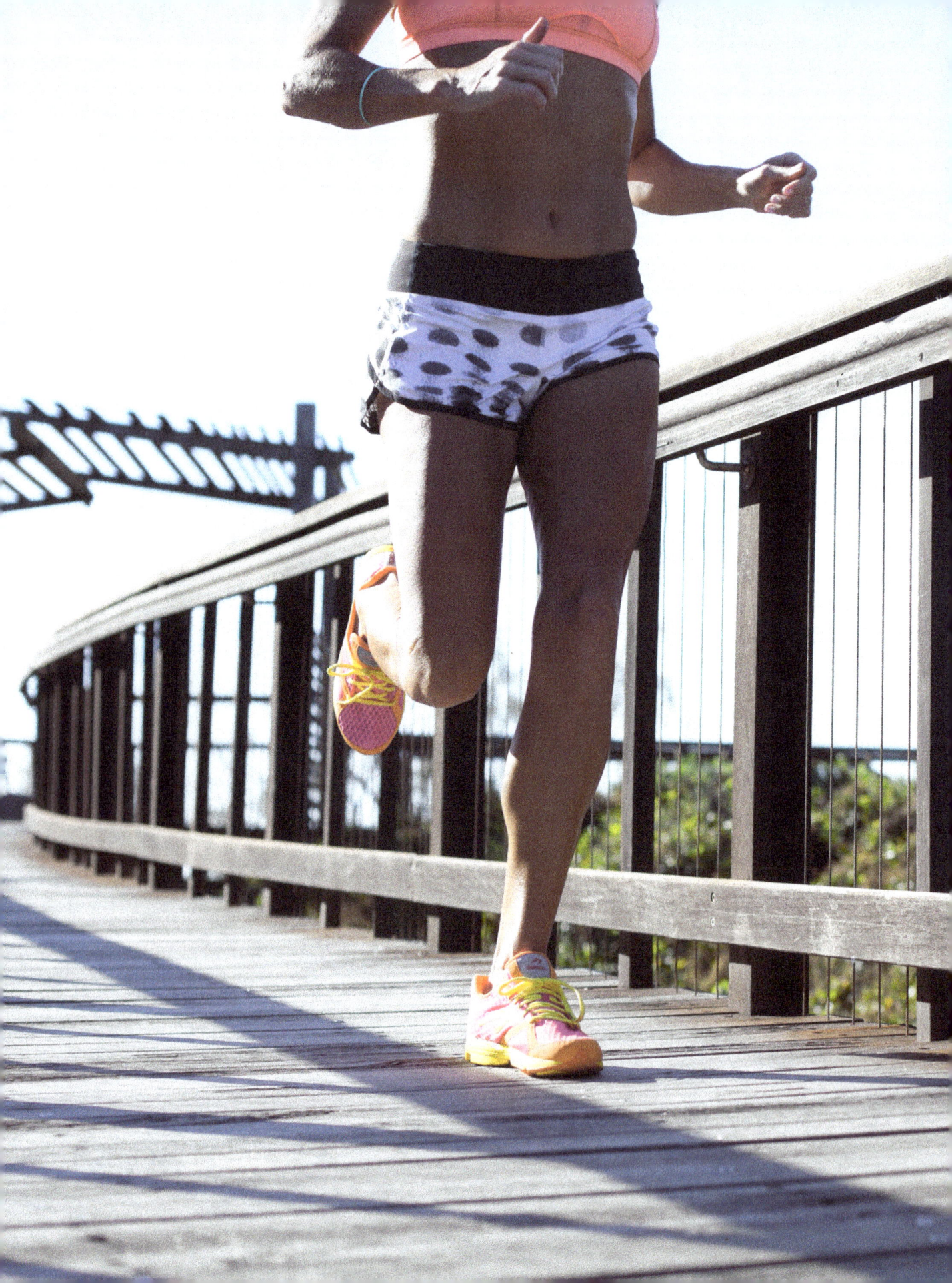

Cardio

Our heart is a muscle and needs the same attention to training and cultivating a healthy lifestyle as the rest of our body. In fact, a healthy heart is vital for a healthy body and mental agility. So, you should think of cardio as essential to your vitality for life program!

The beauty of cardio is that it allows you to workout in new locations and experience different types of cardio, giving your body a change of scenery when it comes to how you train.

Running cardio is different from cycle fitness, for example. Swap the bike for the rowing machine, or the treadmill for a park or hill near you. Jump back in the pool again for some warm-up laps at lunchtime. Maybe even hit a group lesson that focuses on high intensity cardio with motivating music.

2 Common mistakes of cardio training

1. **'Exercising', but not mixing up the heart rate zones.** Remember, your heart is a muscle and it needs to be used at lots of different levels to ensure it stays healthy and active. Cardio health means training in different zones and this means picking up the pace on your morning walks, runs or swims.

2. **Always training at high intensity.** Just like the above point, if you train too hard all the time you won't see long-term results. Ensure you have mixed sessions during your week. Recovery sessions, low and moderate heart rate sessions are great for building endurance.

Did you know?
Your maximum heart rate is 220 minus your age. So you can then workout your heart rate percentages from the calculation.

Zone	Effort	What It Does
1. 50-60%	Low Intensity - Can easily chat away	Beginning of fat burning range if you train consistently here for 20+ minutes.
2. 60-70%	Mod Intensity - Shorter sentences	This is when you start to work your heart as a muscle and push it a bit harder, feeling more out of breath, like you can't talk away as freely as before.
3. 70-85%	High Intensity - Single words	You are working anaerobically now, really pushing your limits.
4. MAX	Can't talk at all	Max exertion, leaving you feeling absolutely spent at the end of the session. Lactic acid builds up and breathing at your max.

For example:
220-38 = 182 (Max heart rate)
154 bpm (beats per minute) is 85% - up tempo
127 bpm is 70% - endurance
109 bpm is 60% low intensity

Cardio interval options:

★ **Beach or park** - use open sprints, stairs and the dunes as your interval sessions.

★ **Limited space (i.e. hotel or apartment)** - use a skipping rope or dynamic warm up exercises.

★ **Indoors** - at the gym, use the treadmill/cross trainer, skipping rope or rowing machine as your interval sessions.

★ **Swimming** - use different tempos with each lap or within laps to pick up the pace or ensure you have a moderate to easy intensity swim as part of recovery for a change.

Core

For long-term health and vitality, it's important to always engage your core. Your abs are your powerhouse: the centre of strength, intuition and energy. Once you learn to connect your core to all your daily activities, you will never look back.

Whether running over rocks, riding a bike, sprinting, lifting weights, reaching for something or even sitting at your desk = your abs are crucial for your ability to live actively and to use the muscles you have to support your skeletal system.

What does engaging your core actually mean?

Have a look around you as you read this: consider your own posture and the posture of others. Are you sitting with your shoulders back and do you feel your abs switched on? Is your back straight?

In simple terms, if I were to ask you to pull your belly button towards your spine you would immediately feel a tightening of your abs and a correlating improvement in your posture. Your back would be straighter, you shoulders would want to go back and your chest would be forward. By this simple act of engaging your core, you have immediately fired up your abs to be active and do their job.

Nikki's fit tip:
- Have total awareness of your core at all times.
- Be sure you have a great technique when working out.
- Focus on form and isolation, to help prevent bigger muscles taking over, such as using your legs or back to help.

Engaging you core

Ab work is not about bouts of sit-ups or crunches in the gym. It is about a daily, hourly, consistent practice of body awareness; when you know you can engage your abs and use your core in ALL your activities.

Try it out while you are presenting to a group or colleagues; stand on one leg while you are brushing your teeth; pull your belly button to your spine to add balance; walk tall and with purpose; press lightly on your abs before you commence a run or exercise to remind those muscles they are needed; and remind yourself to activate them in all that you do.

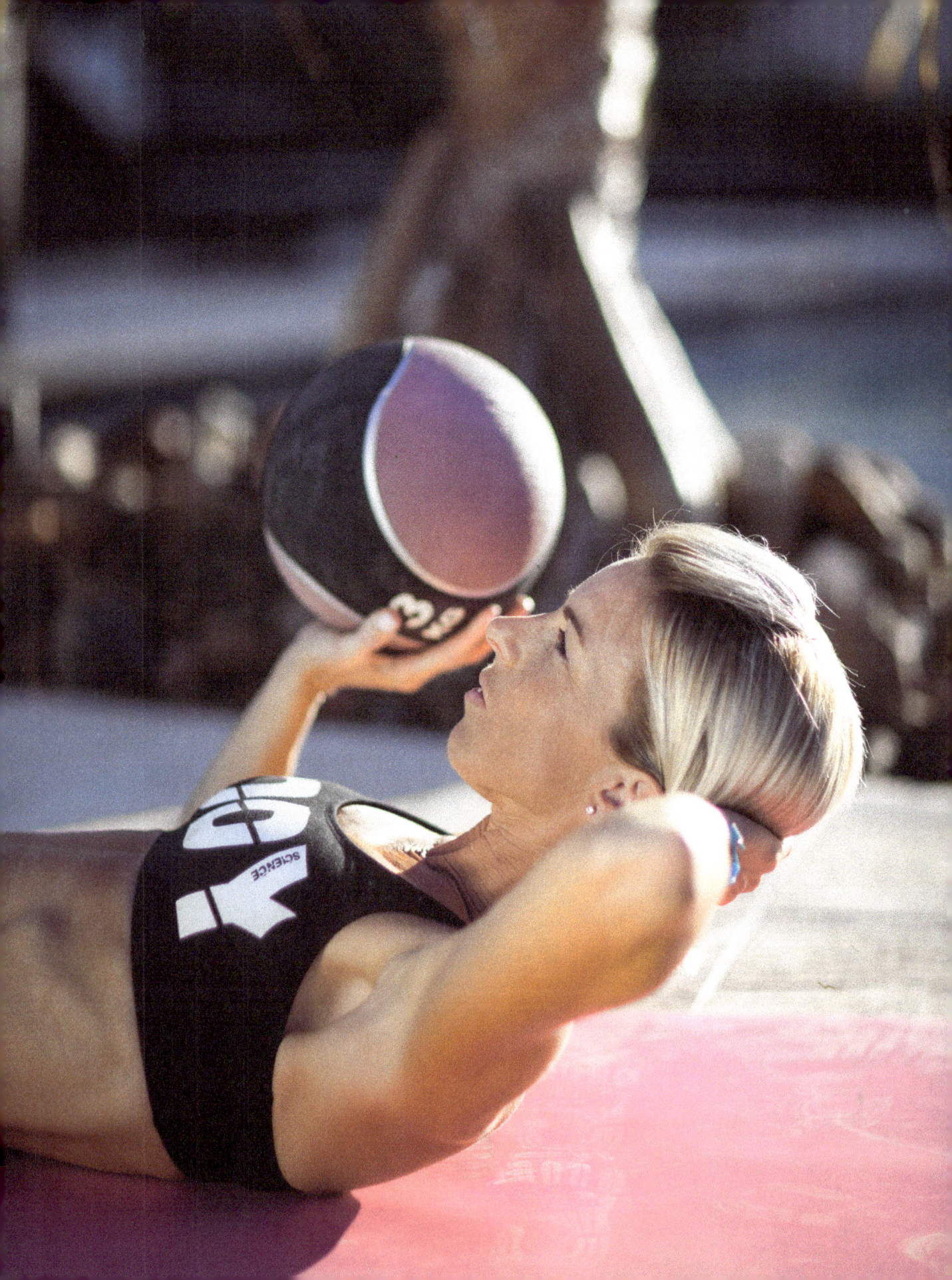

You will be surprised at the results from using your abs daily with everything you do. Those rows of incredible small and functional muscles are designed to keep us upright, to keep us centred and to help us navigate our way through physical and mental challenges.

Once you learn to connect your core to all your daily activities you will never look back. Your abs are crucial for your ability to live actively and use the muscles you have to support your skeletal system, whether you're running over rocks, riding a bike, sprinting, lifting weights, reaching for something or even sitting at your desk.

5 Fun ways to get started:
★ Put a sticky note on your laptop that says "Belly Button To Spine" or quite simply "ABS"
★ Squeeze your abs when you reach out to shake someone's hand, to reach for something or to do a simple action even at your desk
★ Stand on one leg and alternate this to engage your core muscles while cooking or brushing your teeth or even making the kids' lunches
★ Sit up straight at your desk or the board table during a meeting, and even while driving
★ Walk tall and be aware of your abs as you are walking around

Back to basics
Think you know how to do basic crunches? Think again: it is all about technique and the truth is, most people get it wrong. Your head is actually the heaviest part of your body and it should be supported by your hands completely, with no tension in your neck at all.

For more on perfecting crunches, visit www.thevitalitycoach.com.au or watch the free videos on my YOUTUBE channel VitalityCoachTV

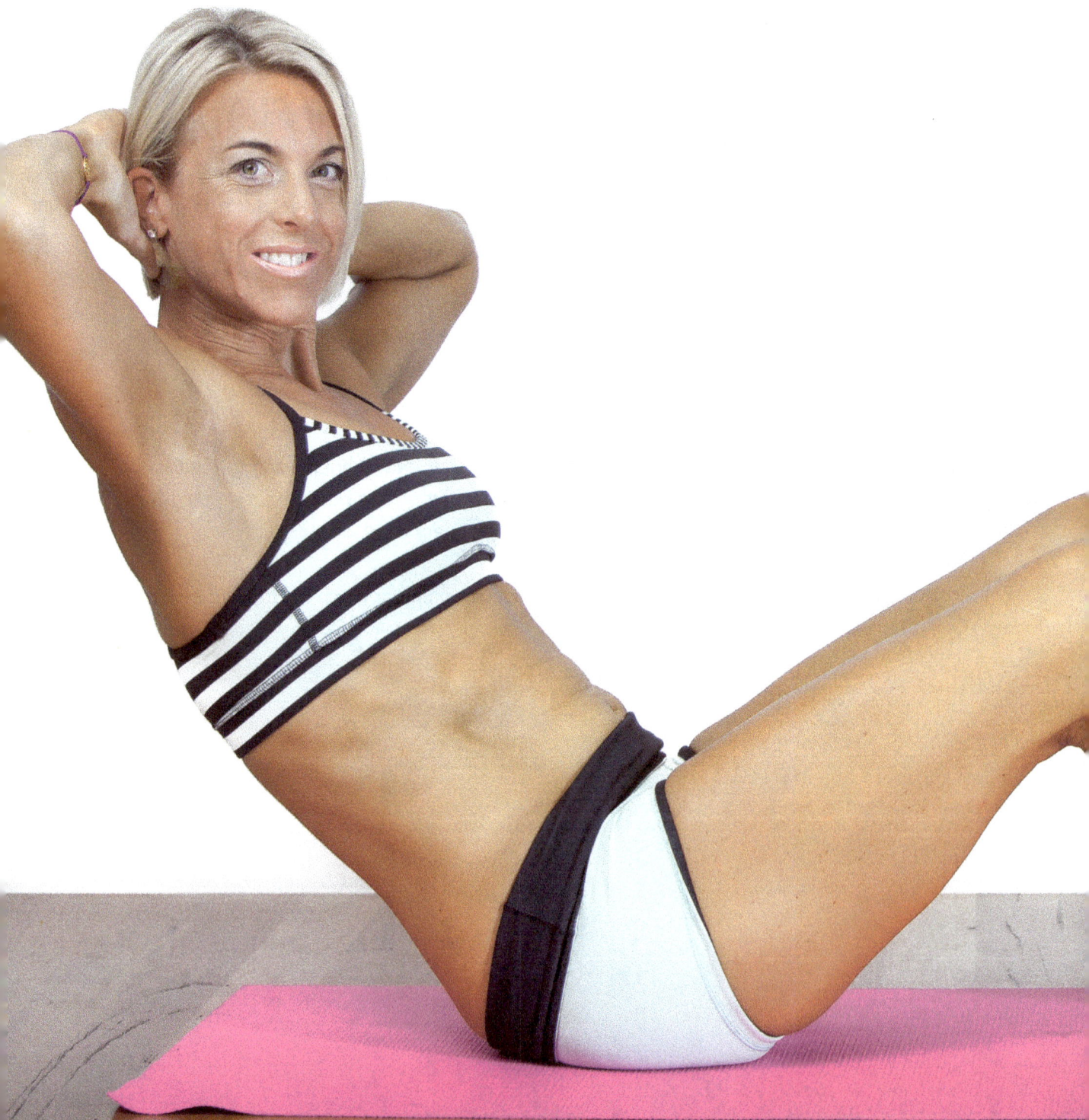

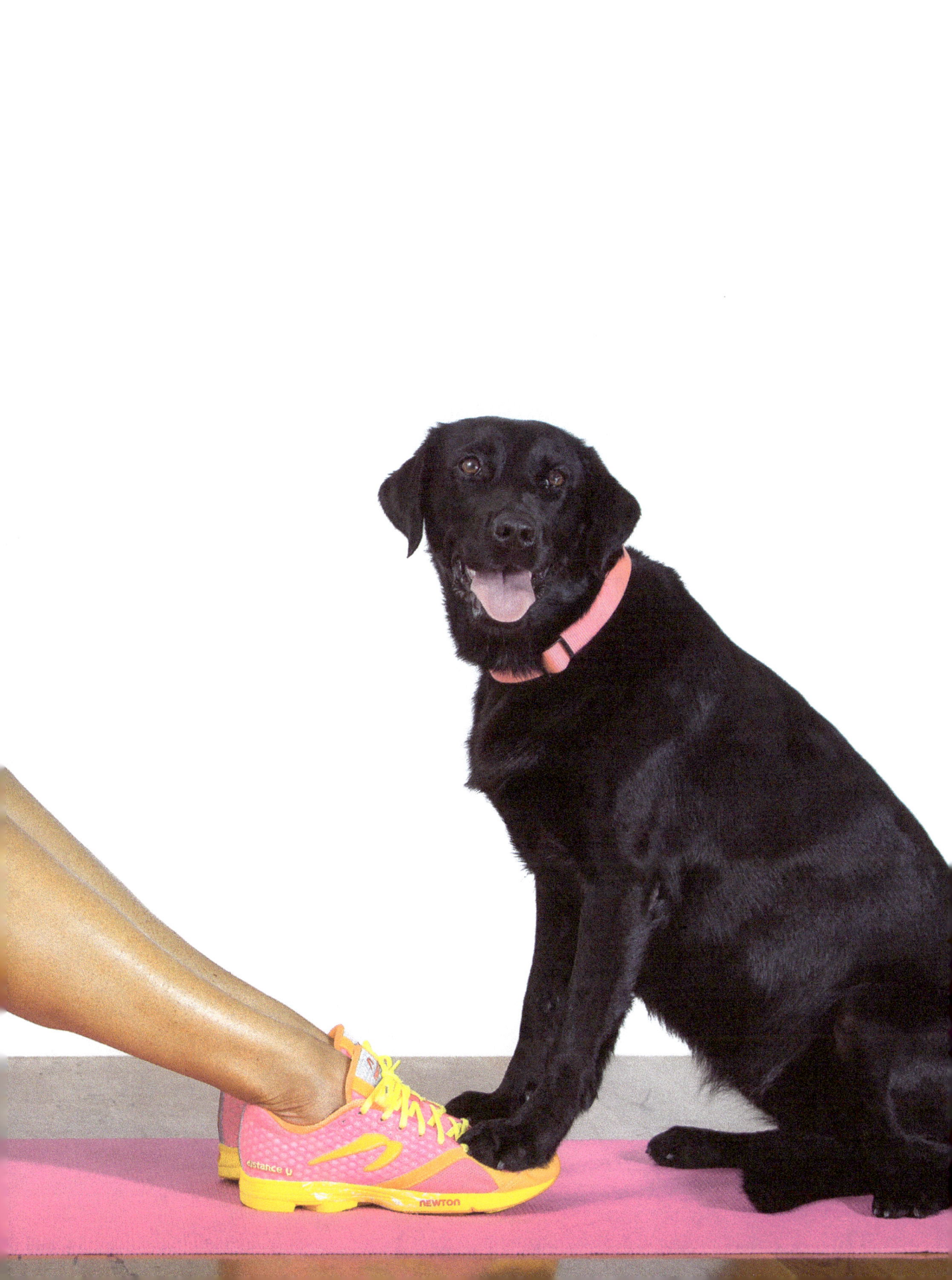

Getting fit with your dog

There is no better example of nature being used as a gym than when watching your dog run around and play.

I've always grown up with dogs, and it s been a firm directive in our family that a happy pet is a healthy pet. That always meant plenty of fresh air, nutritious food and getting out and about for some daily exercise – rain, hail or shine.

Like people, every dog is different. They each come in different shapes, sizes, breeds, with varying personalities and some pre-dispositions.

Here are a few factors to consider:

PUPPIES: Listen to the vet to ensure you're not running your dog while their bones develop. In most cases this is up to 2 years of age and certainly no stairs in the early months as well.

SMALL DOGS: If you have a tiny dog with short legs it s not the best idea to take them for a long walk or run. Boxers, bulldogs and dogs with shorter snouts can have more difficulty breathing than other breeds with longer noses.

MID-SIZE DOGS: If you have a mid-size dog that is heavily built and all muscle, they are more suited to interval short runs than long endurance activities.

TALL/LARGE DOGS: Longer leg/body dogs such as labradors, border collies, weimaraner and mastiffs all love to run and have the stamina. However, you need to build up their fitness slowly. Just like getting fit yourself, your dog needs time to acclimatise to a new routine.

3 Canine-ready workouts

1. Interval sessions and shuttle runs:

Incorporate small walk/runs with shuttle runs, stairs and games where you are both doing intervals, and your dog runs beside you. It s fun, engaging and you can create a game for your dog and provide anaerobic exercise, toning and fun for you too.

2. The "athletic dog" workout:

5km runs are a great distance for dogs – anything longer and you need to make sure you worked with your dog over time to build up the distance. Start out with run/walks and then build from there. Take your dog trail running or along the beach.

3. Yoga time:

Whenever I pull my yoga mat out, Roxy always wants to sit on it. Stretching and functional fitness is fun with your dog if you incorporate them. Push-ups with your dog in the front is fun and it brings a whole new meaning to 'downward dog

Don't be afraid to call your vet to ensure you have some general rules on what type of exercise best suits your dog breed and will prevent injury. Pay attention to this as your four-legged training buddy will most likely soldier through any kind of pain, so you need to be considerate and tailor your workouts for them.

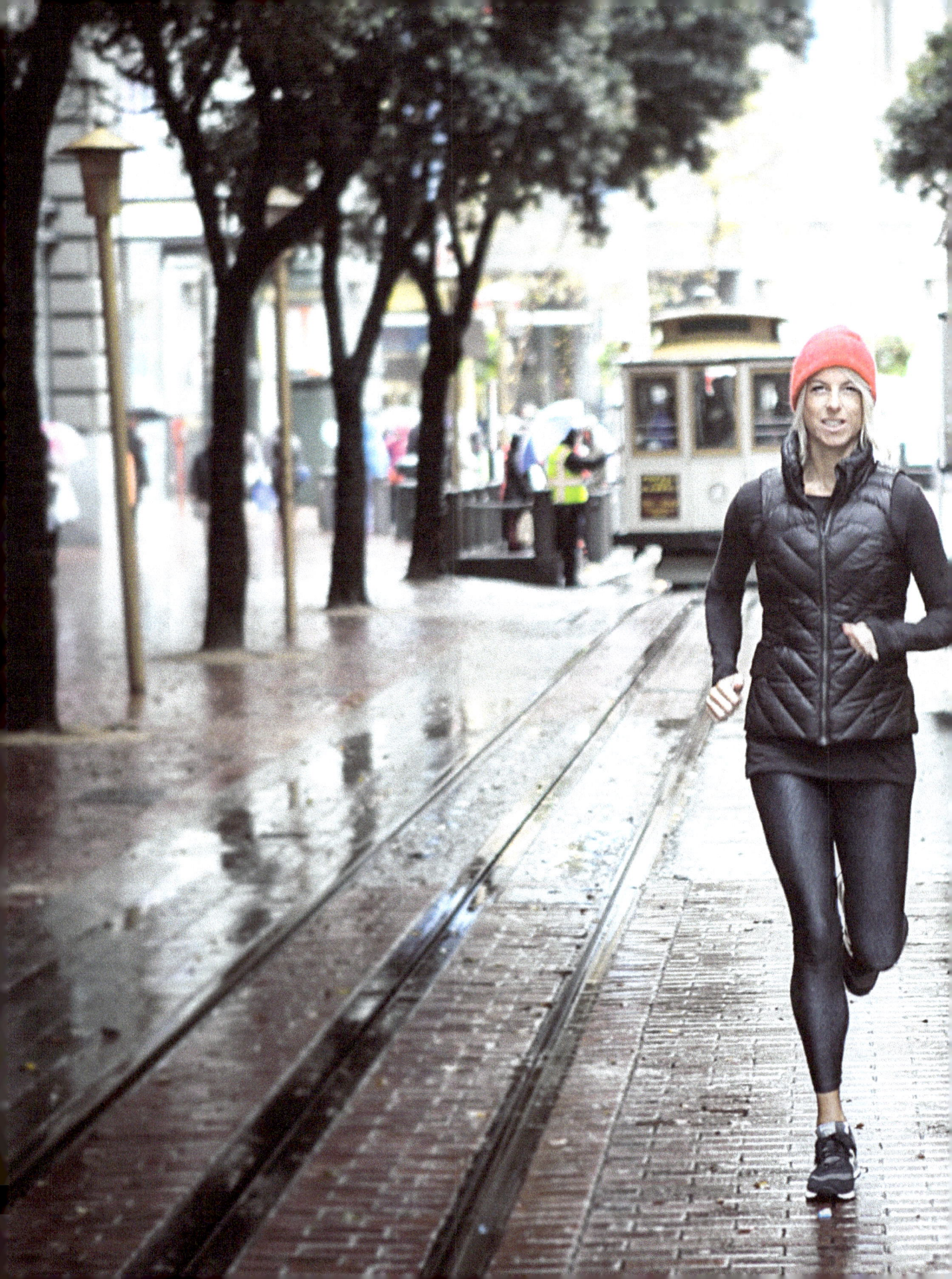

POWELL AND MARKET

HYDE AND BEACH
FISHERMANS WHARF

15

Travel fitness

Whether you're spending a week at the beach, seeing the sights in NYC, travelling interstate on business or you're heading off on an escape to the countryside, there are always ways you can integrate fitness into your travel schedule.

It's actually easier than you may think to take your 'gym' with you, by using body weight exercises and packing some basic lightweight items and a pair of running shoes.

A great place to start is to explore where you are on foot or by bike – simply swap your heels or dress shoes for trainers and get to know your new surroundings. Exploring the city before everything opens is the perfect way to get your bearings.

If you're staying at a big resort, you can ask to borrow a yoga mat, otherwise just put on your shoes and head out the door to explore. The world is your oyster!

When time is not on your side, there are still a number of short yet powerful workouts you can unleash (see opposite page). That said, if you are tired, then listen to your body: rest, relax and eat healthily to recharge and rejuvenate. The ultimate aim is to find exercise while you are away that seamlessly fits into your day, and creates a nice moment to switch off and a different way to see the environment you are in.

Nikki's fit tip:
I am on the road every week with early starts and late finishes, but that never stops me from getting my fit-fix. If you pack your running shoes and one or two fitness-ready outfits, you're always good to go. If I'm going for any longer than a weekend, I also pack CrankIT straps and a skipping rope.

6 Travel-friendly workouts:

15 Minute Express Session: Quick walk or jog followed by a super set of 25 push ups, 25 crunches, 25 triceps dips and 25 prisoner squats. Finish with three yoga poses to stretch.

Skip your way fit: A skipping rope will roll up and fit in your shoe. Skip as a warm up and cool down at different tempos, then add your core work and body weight exercises in between. You'll be surprised how effective skipping is for agility and cardio condition.

Use the on-site gym or pool: Research where you are staying and find out what facilities they have onsite. Pack your swim goggles and squeeze in a few laps between dinners and other activities.

Pack suspension straps: Take your gym with you with some suspension straps. I always take these on trips of four days or more and it ensures I can train on the spot for just 15 minutes a day, or longer combined with cardio.

Use nature as your gym: Embrace the surroundings. If you're on an island paradise or beach holiday, then head to the water for your workouts. In the countryside or even in a city that has amazing parks, head out to explore by hiking, running, walking, biking or even look at horse riding for a more adventurous twist.

★

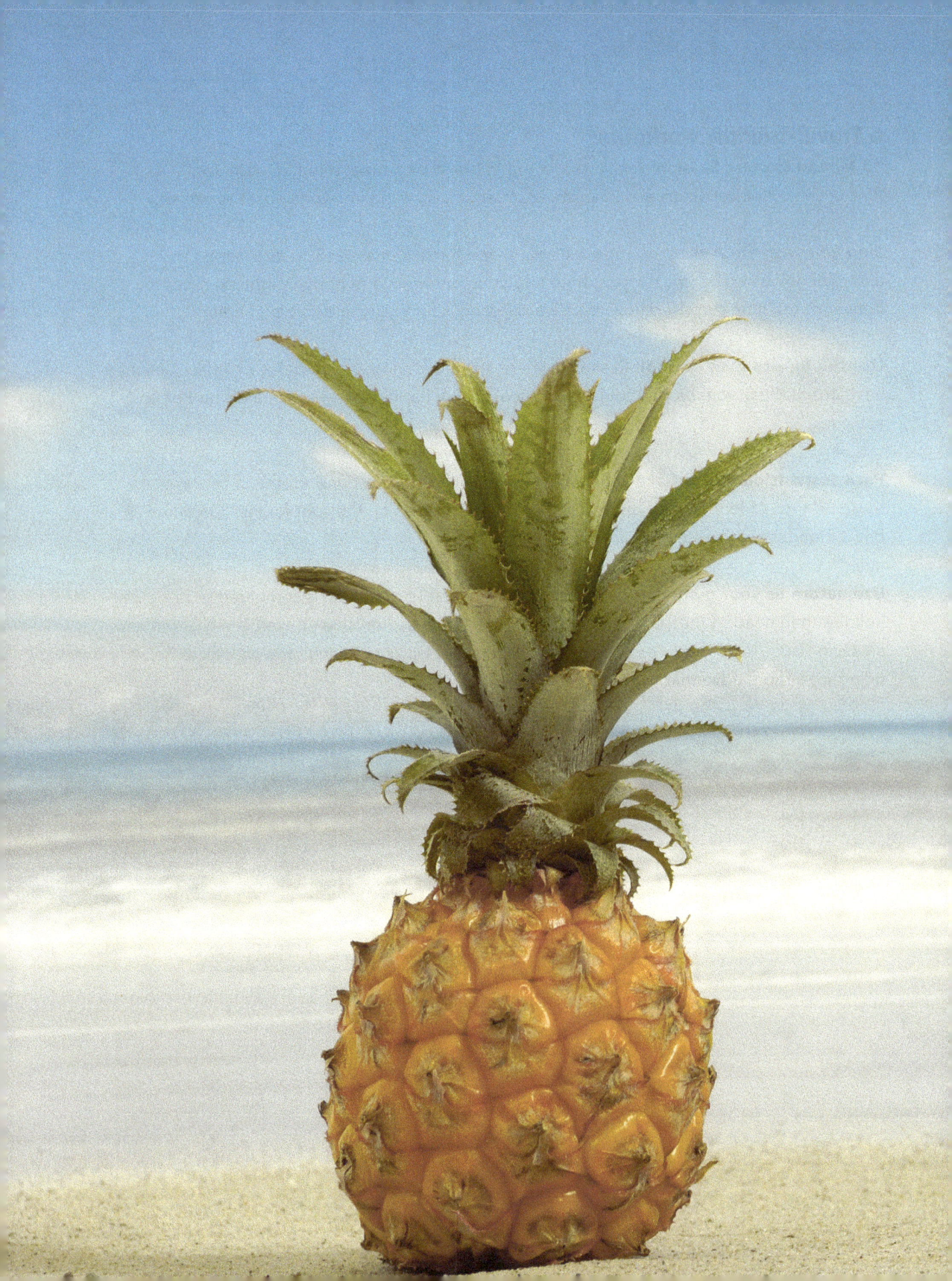

CHAPTER THREE: FRESH FOOD

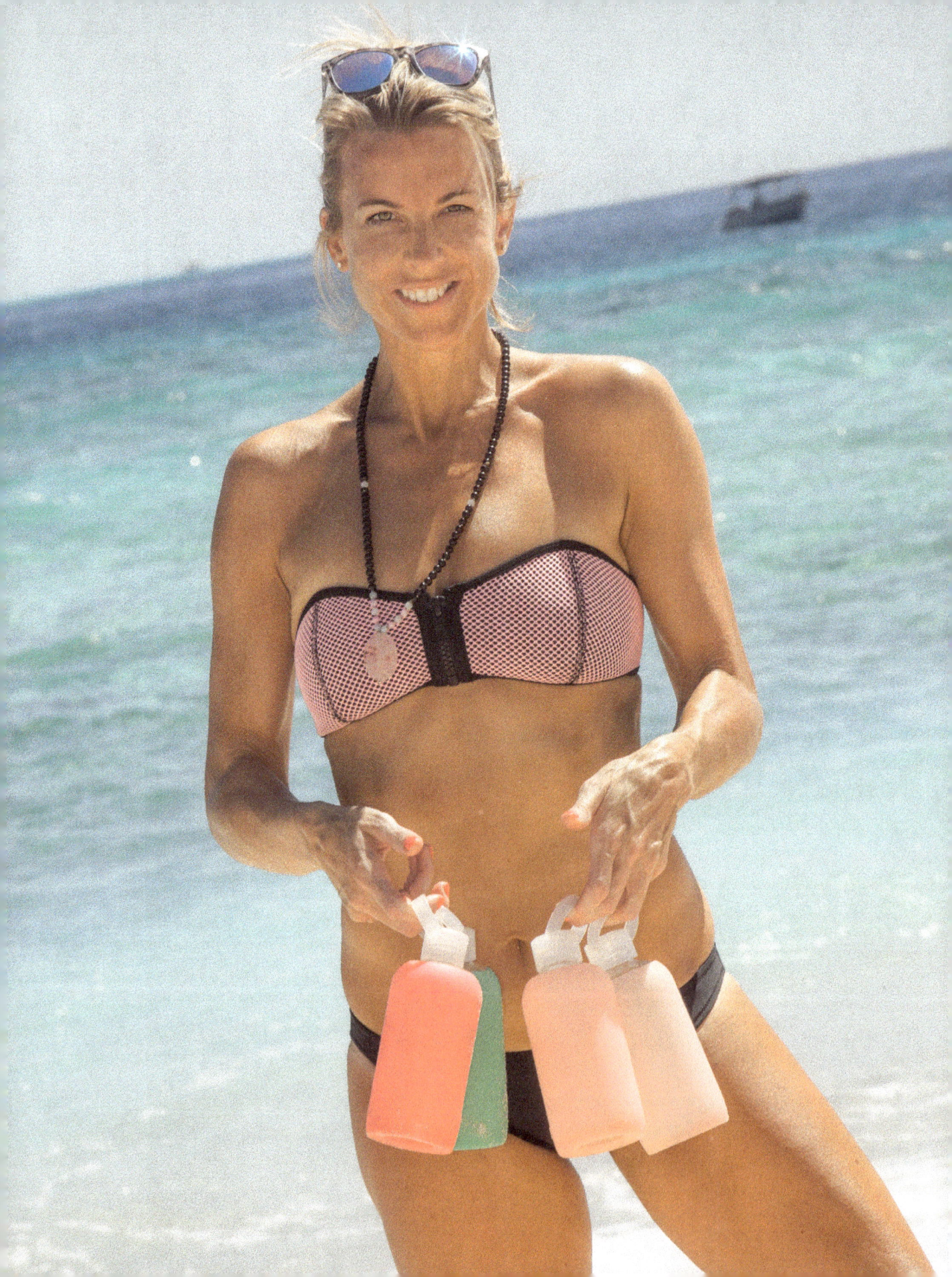

Your mental wellbeing and mood is fundamentally connected to what you eat and drink, so to feel your best, you need to fuel your body with the best. The question is, what does that mean? I've had some really interesting conversations with smart, savvy people who have lost their way on the food and fitness map. Their main complaint is often the same: it's all so confusing.

Sugar free, dairy free, wheat free, gluten free, everything free… Low fat, high protein, low carb, intense cardio. You name it, it's out there. And it claims to be "the solution" to your health concerns. But unless we look at the big picture, we won't ever achieve total health.

My motto is simple: for optimal health you need fresh food and fitness, without turning your life upside down.

Get back to basics

In a cluttered health and fitness market promoting fast weight loss, rapid muscle gain, six-pack abs and anytime 24/7 gym memberships, why is it that our obesity rates are on the increase?

In my view, it's because we've forgotten to live the basics: fresh food, fresh air, plenty of sleep and doing what you love.

In order to get the body you want, you need to get off autopilot, stop spending money on quick fixes and get back to the chopping board with some fresh ingredients that will nourish your senses and your soul.

In other words, you need to get back to basics.

Remember:

- ★ The closer food is to its natural source, the better it is for you.
- ★ If you can't pronounce the ingredient or it has a number, then you can be pretty sure your body is not designed to digest it.
- ★ Our bodies are built to work with nature: the combination of fibre, vitamins, nutrients, carbs, fats and proteins in plants and natural produce are all designed to work in harmony. Strip them apart, and you're not getting the whole picture.

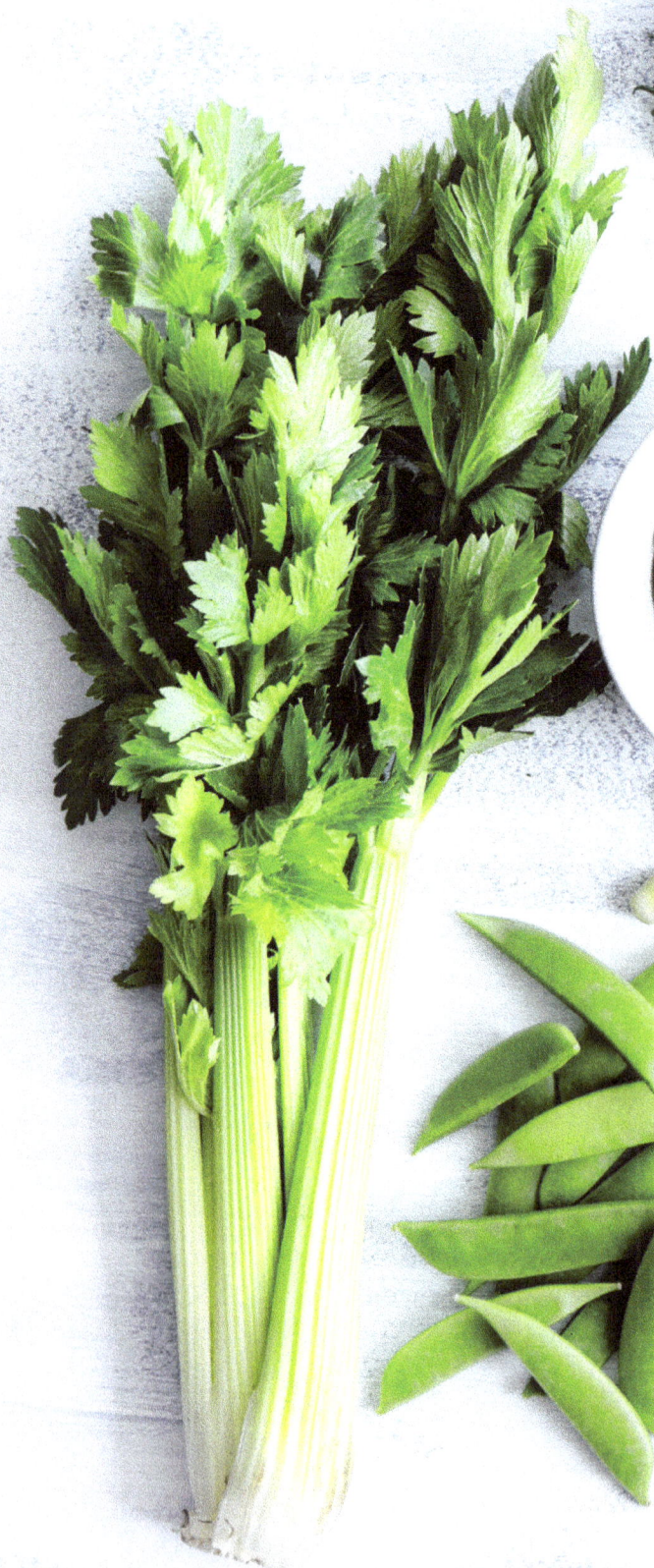

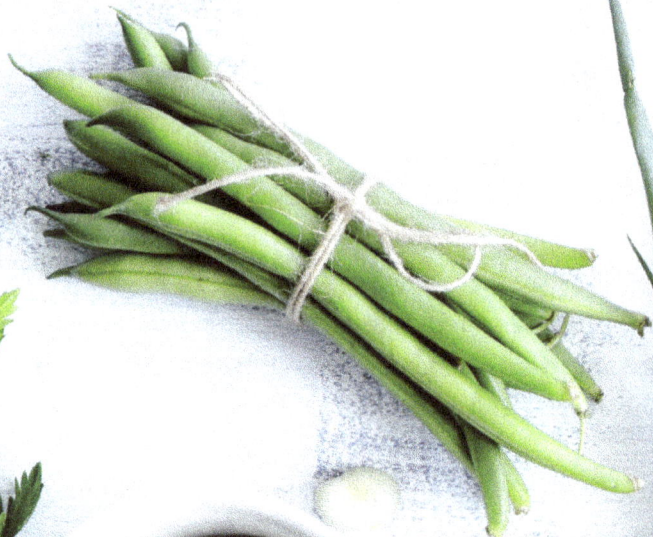

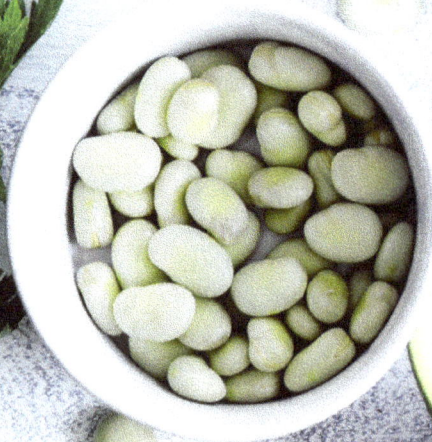

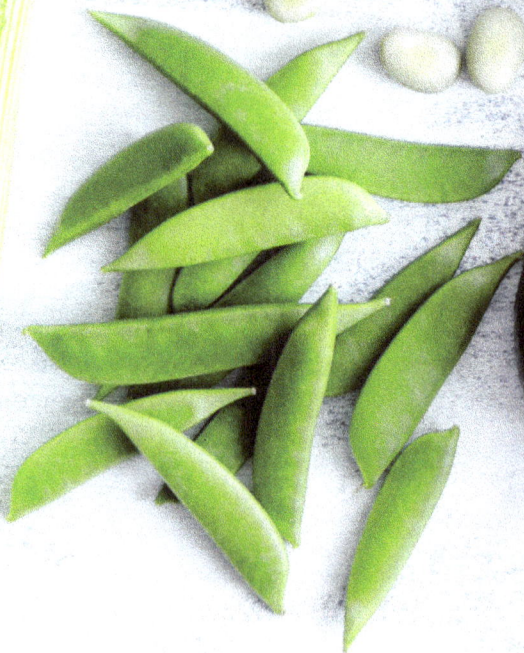

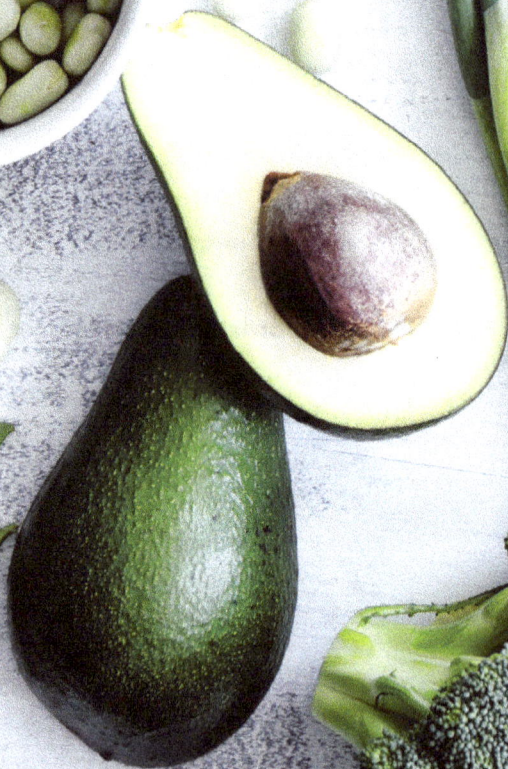

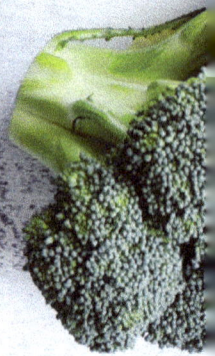

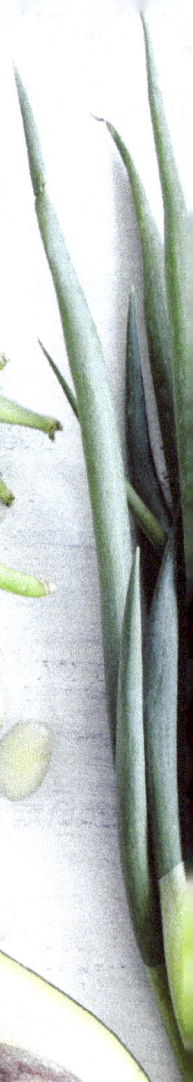

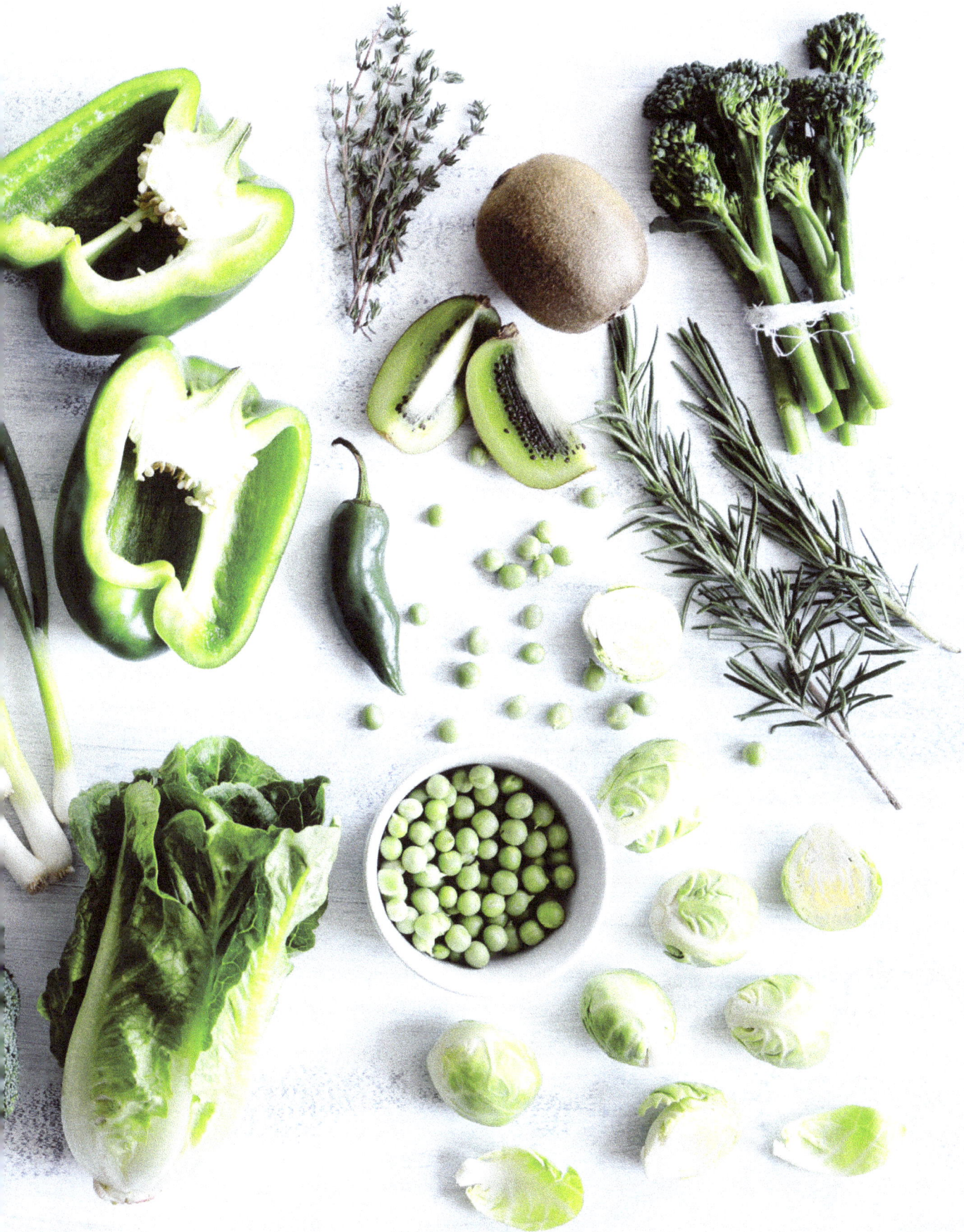

Fast track to healthy habits

When you fill up on foods that contain a lot of artificial sweeteners, such as fizzy drinks, crisps and ready-made snacks, you are really filling up on empty calories. They contain plenty of calories but still leave you wanting more, driving your desire for more of these kinds of foods.

But that's not the worst of it: the problem for your body is that it doesn't know how to process a lot of the foreign, man-made "food" you ingest, which can cause all sorts of health issues, immediately and down the track.

The best thing you can do to fast track your journey towards embracing healthier habits is to fuel yourself with delicious but healthy foods that provide energy and nutrients. Detoxing from a lifetime of packed and processed food takes time, but the rewards are endless.

Basic food rules to live by:

1. **Upgrade your breakfast** - Swap fried eggs and bacon for poached/boiled eggs with tomato, spinach and beans.
2. **Rein in red meat** - Minimising meat helps to reduce low-grade inflammation and lower risk of heart disease and diabetes.
3. **Boost fibre intake** - When you replace all or part of the meat portion in a recipe with legumes or extra vegetables, you increase fibre while reducing fat.
4. **Reduce the portion size of meals** - And remember, the meat portion should be smaller than your palm.
5. **Eat good carbohydrates** - Brown rice, quinoa or legumes such as beans and lentils will increase fibre, keep you full and cleanse your body.
6. **Perfect your plate** - Aim for 1/2 of your plate to be vegetables, 1/4 wholegrain carbohydrate, and 1/4 lean meat, eggs, seafood or cheese.
7. **Snack smart** - Try two pieces of fruit, two hard-boiled eggs, a protein shake, a small handful of nuts or even water
8. **Slow down** - Eating slowly and making the effort to put down your cutlery between bites helps your body register that you're filling up. It takes time for the signals to reach your brain!
9. **Hydrate** - great quality water is the elixir to a healthy body inside and out. Really make a conscious effort to drink at least 10 glasses of water a day or I prefer to think in 1l bottles – at east 2 of those.

Daily Dose

Making sure you have all the right ingredients is essential, or you'll sabotage your efforts before you've even begun. The following guideline will help you prepare a daily meal plan that leaves you feeling satiated and satisfied.

FAT:

A certain amount of natural, essential fats are crucial to keep your body in tip-top condition. Aim to get your requirements from foods such as avocado, nuts, fish and seeds, rather than from fried or processed foods that often contain low quality vegetable oils and trans fats.

FIBRE:

Increasing the amount of whole grains, vegetables, fruits and beans you eat will increase your fibre intake. Fibre is essential for great digestion, healthy gut bacteria, feeling full and eliminating waste and toxins.

MINERALS:

Mineral-rich foods are truly essential in your daily diet. Magnesium, zinc, calcium and potassium are some of the minerals you need to aid, repair and develop a strong immune system.

PROTEIN:

Something of a wonder-food, protein stabilises your blood sugar, stimulates lean muscle, builds the immune system and helps the body recover and repair: in other words, it's essential. The trick is not to overdo it. Include protein in small serves throughout the day to stave off hunger and help your body absorb and utilise the amino acids most effectively. Adding a few scoops of natural protein powder to a smoothie, or selecting lean sources of grass-fed beef, organic chicken, non-farmed fish or legumes are just some ways you can fortify your diet with protein.

The no diet rule
It's easy to underestimate the journey from average eating patterns to having a balanced healthy lifestyle. When you embrace the 'fresh is best' philosophy, you will find yourself sourcing, tasting and enjoying the best possible fuel for your body.

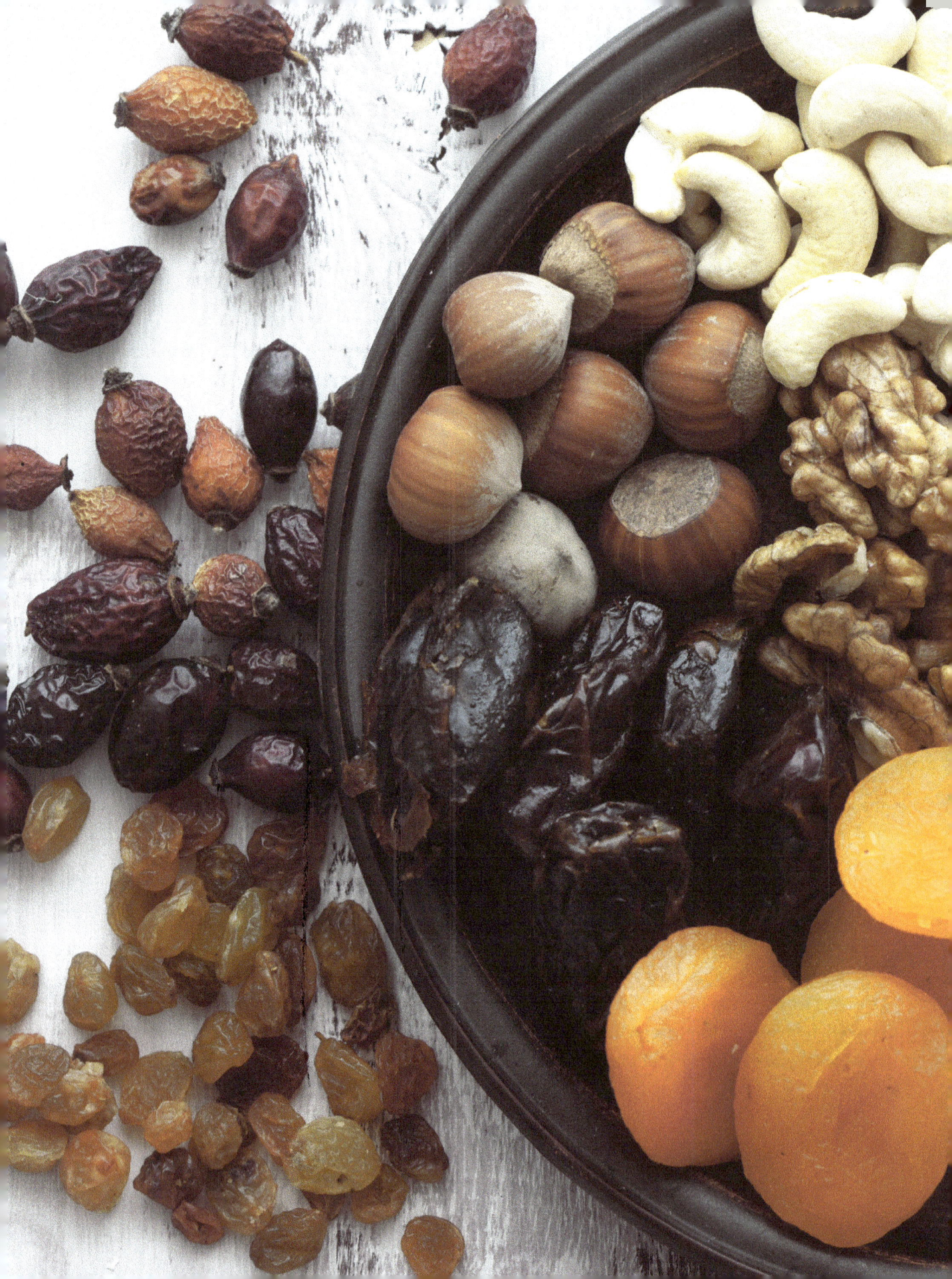

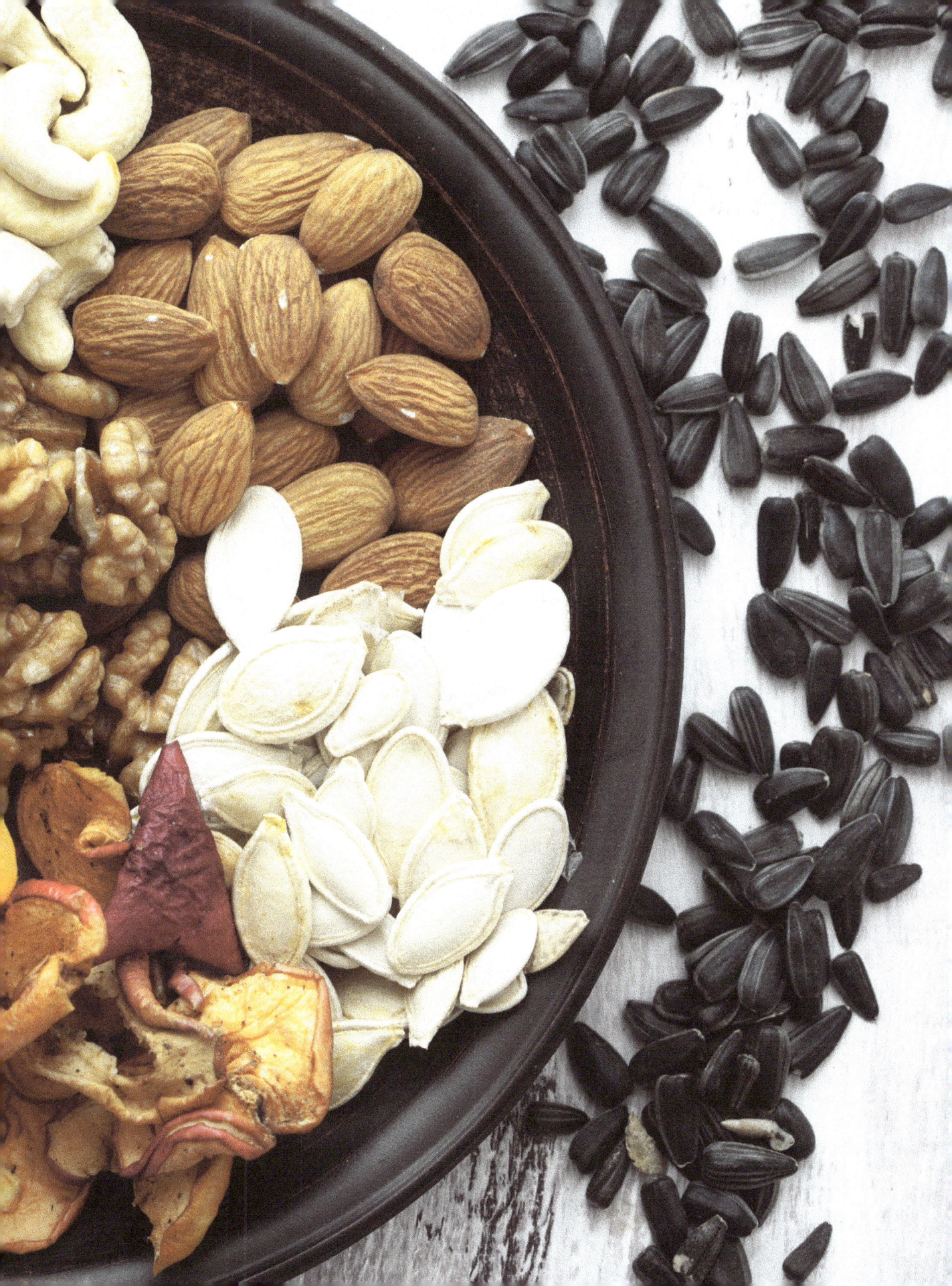

Foods containing roughly 20g of protein:

70g chicken breast
65g beef
3 large eggs
1 cup firm tofu
1.5 cups lentils (1 large tin)
1/2 cup pumpkin seeds
1 cup nuts (note: due to high energy value, nuts should be eaten in small amounts only)
500g or 2 cups natural good quality yoghurt
1 serve tuna

Here are some "side effects" of healthy eating. Be warned: they can be addictive...

- ★ Increased metabolism
- ★ Better sleep patterns
- ★ Feeling fitter, faster and stronger
- ★ Clearer thinking
- ★ Improved mobility and strength
- ★ Increased mindfulness
- ★ Frequent jumping about with unbounded energy
- ★ Smiling... a lot!
- ★ Clear skin
- ★ Shiny hair
- ★ Happy demeanour
- ★ The ability to get out of bed in the morning without a forklift

Infecting others with your positivity (note that not everyone is keen on this infectious enthusiasm...)

Myth Busting

★ Carbs are not evil: Just make sure you opt for high fibre, low GI (glycaemic index) options which will release energy slowly.

★ Don't limit yourself: Make sure you eat enough – it's about eating the right kind of calories, not avoiding them altogether.

★ Positive lifestyle choices will create long-term benefits and balance: Find the freshest ingredients you can as a way to give your body extra vitamins

How to ditch unhealthy snacks?

Replace junk food and high sugary fixes with a healthy stack of snacks you have on hand. Each week, pre-pack for your desk, handbag or gym bag a mix of the following:

★ A bag of nuts and seeds: dry roast them for extra flavour.

★ Protein bar without artificial colourings or preservatives.

★ Fresh fruit and crunchy veggie sticks.

★ Natural nut butter you can leave in the fridge at work.

★ Homemade bliss balls.

★ Plenty of filtered water

Buying Organic: What to Look For

If you buy organic food, it will be healthier and better for you – right? In a general sense, this is true – although you need to know that not all organic labelled products are equal.

In a nutshell, organic produce and other ingredients used in organic products are grown without the use of pesticides, synthetic fertilisers, sewage sludge, genetically modified organisms, or ionising radiation. This includes animals that produce meat, poultry, eggs, and dairy products, who do not take antibiotics or growth hormones.

The Australian Certified Organics group go one step further and talk about not only the source, but how products are prepared, including to some degree how well live animals are treated. They mention, "The whole system is linked: Soil. Plants. Animals. Food. People. Environment".

FRESH FOOD ★ . . . .

Food and produce certified organic have varying degrees of guidelines they need to reach in order to bear the "organic" tag. Some companies use the 'organic' label but the truth is, if you really dived into their ingredients, farming and source, the organic component is minimal at best. They may have only a certain percentage of ingredients that are organic to ensure they meet the label standards.

Organic breakdown

The US Department of Agriculture has identified three categories of labelling organic products:

★ **100% Organic:** Made with 100% organic ingredients.
★ **Organic:** Made with at least 95% organic ingredients.
★ **Made With Organic Ingredients:** Made with a minimum of 70% organic ingredients with strict restrictions on the remaining 30%, including no genetically modified organisms.

How can you tell you are buying organic?

In Australia, the majority of organic products sold carry the Australian Certified Organic BUD Logo. You will see the BUD on products ranging from apples to baby food, coffee to liquorice, clothing to cosmetics. In the US there is also a certified organic label, which is how you can recognise that the product has been certified according to USDA standards.

Why does organic cost more?

In most countries, organic farmers and sustainable factories are not given the extra government or industry subsidies like their volume-driven, factory farming counterparts. This gravely affects the numbers of farmers, producers and manufacturers that try to adhere to a true organic philosophy, as they are working against the system that supports mass production, volume of product and transportation. To be truly organic, it also means that the manufacturing process cannot be mixed with any non-organic ingredients, so this means a separate plant or production line as well.

82

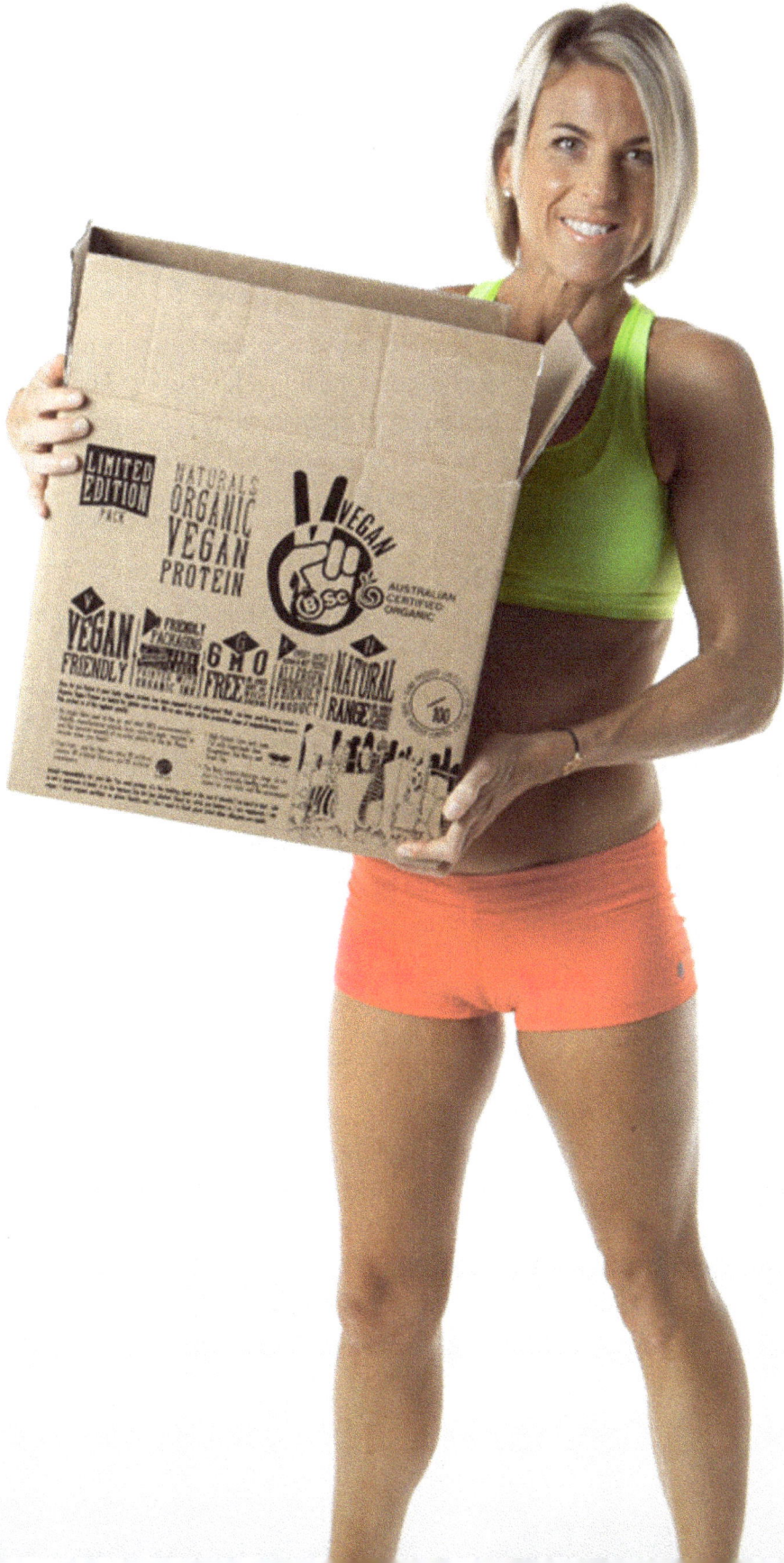

LIMITED EDITION PACK

NATURALS
ORGANIC
VEGAN
PROTEIN

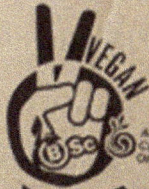

VEGAN

BSc

AUSTRALIAN CERTIFIED ORGANIC

VEGAN FRIENDLY

FRIENDLY PACKAGING

GMO FREE

ALLERGEN FRIENDLY PRODUCT

NATURAL RANGE

Conscious living

So you want to do all the right things: eat fresh, whole foods; buy local, cruelty-free products; eat organic and avoid mass-produced products. Plus, you want to make sure that you are as fit and healthy as possible.

But how can you do all of this without turning your life upside down?

The truth is, the pursuit of conscious living is not for those who want the easy road. It's for those who want to make a difference in their lives now, and the future for those to come. And, it doesn't have to be so complicated. Making a commitment to accountability in every decision you make, not simply 'consuming' products and information on autopilot and instead, being informed, interested and intrigued about what foods you are eating and where they come from.

My top tips for conscious living:
★ **Get informed:** do your research, find out about the terms 'food miles' and 'cruelty free',
★ **Buy local:** source local suppliers and support small business in your area. Get to know your butcher, green grocer and fish monger – you'll get better service, minimise your food miles and learn loads!
★ **Reduce your meat consumption:** meat, especially red, is an inefficient way to produce protein, or ensure you are not having red meat at every meal and do your research on finding really great quality sustainably raised and produced meats – avoid fast packed, volume supermarket meats that are from big farms. A great way is to buy your meats and fish from the local markets each week – ensuring they are fresh, you can ask the right questions and help support the local farmers and community. Environmentally speaking, you're better off choosing local farmed produce, legumes, nuts, seeds, free range eggs and grains. It's cheaper in the long run and so much better for you.

Healthy day in snapshot
★ Start the day with your WakeUp Workout™ then a glass of water with fresh lemon juice upon waking (warm in winter, cool in summer).

Breakfast for getting back to basics
★ Natural, un-toasted muesli – sugar free with low fat yoghurt. Add a serve of protein powder to your yoghurt to help keep you feeling full for longer.

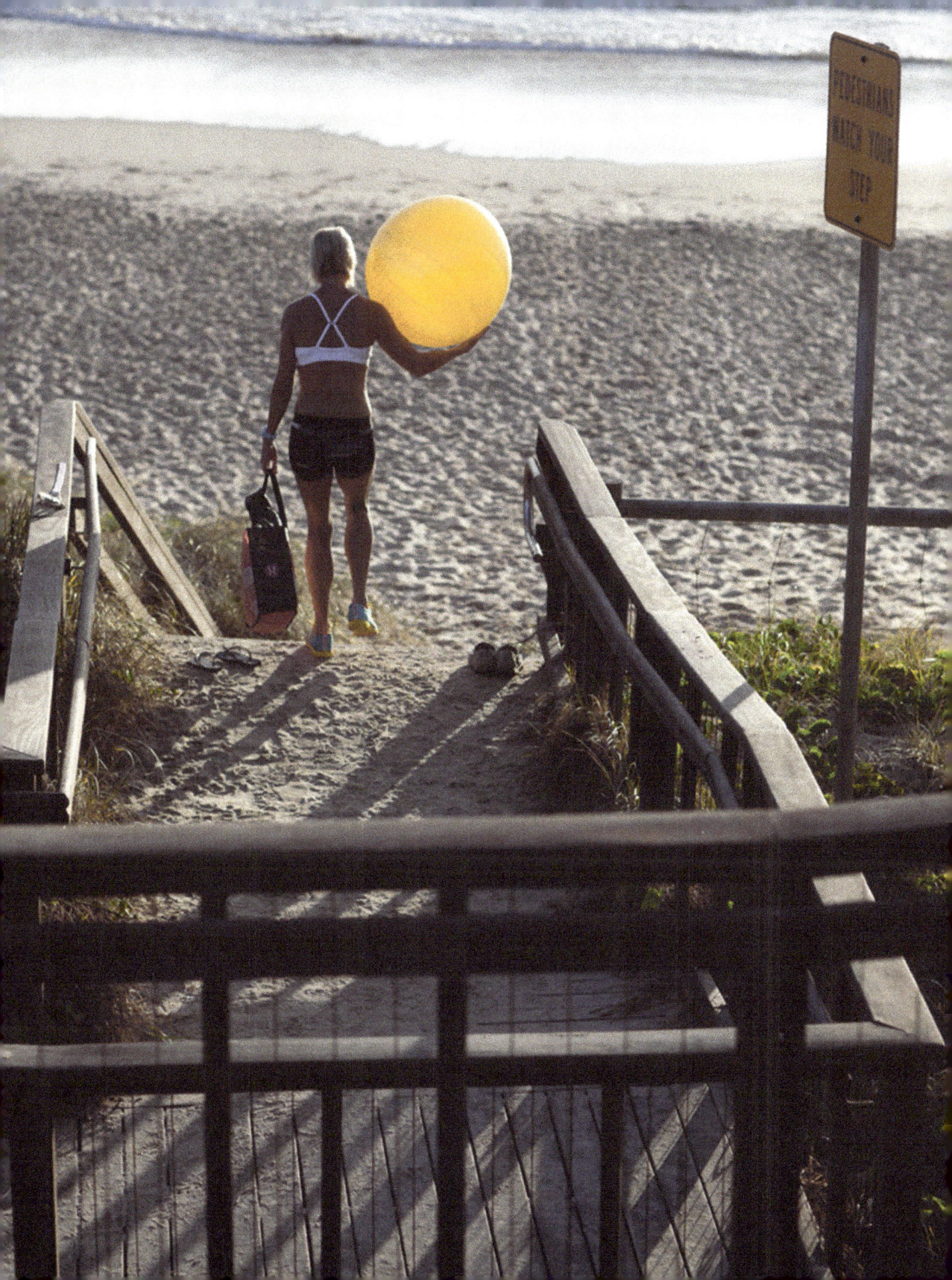

- ★ Smoothie with frozen berries, 1 serve protein powder, 1 tsp spirulina or Vital Greens and coconut water or almond milk.
- ★ Omelette or scrambled eggs with chopped tomatoes, fresh herbs, onion, spinach and mushrooms
- ★ Dark rye toast with almond butter and half a banana, if you're in a rush.

Mid morning and mid afternoon snacks

- ★ Fruit and whole grain peanut butter sandwich on dark or high-fibre bread.
- ★ Handful of almonds.
- ★ Brookfarm Walkabout Mix snack packs homemade trail mix.
- ★ Protein shake or small protein bar.
- ★ Hard-boiled egg.
- ★ 1/2 avocado on two grainy crackers.

Dinner

- ★ Grilled salmon steak with spinach and herb salad, topped with nuts and feta cheese.
- ★ Tofu stir-fry with brown rice and vegetables.
- ★ Roast vegetable and quinoa salad with spinach, fresh herbs and lemon juice.
- ★ Home made pizzas with fresh seafood and a little cheese topped with rocket (I use gluten free bases).
- ★ Vegetable soup – make a big batch and put extra in the freezer.

Evening snacks

- ★ Instead of dessert, make a small protein-rich shake with half a banana and half a cup frozen berries, chia seeds and natural protein powder. Make a smaller portion than you would other times of the day and avoid adding dairy or heavy products - I use coconut water instead.
- ★ Berries or mango topped with dollop of natural or Greek yoghurt.
- ★ Nut butter on sliced apple.
- ★ Green tea

My 3 fresh food mantras:

1. Look at fresh markets and the fresh food aisle in your supermarket as the 'vitamin and mineral' aisle.
2. Choose plenty of colourful fruits and vegetables. More colours means more variety of nutrients
3. Look at the whole picture of your entire week, not just meal-by-meal.

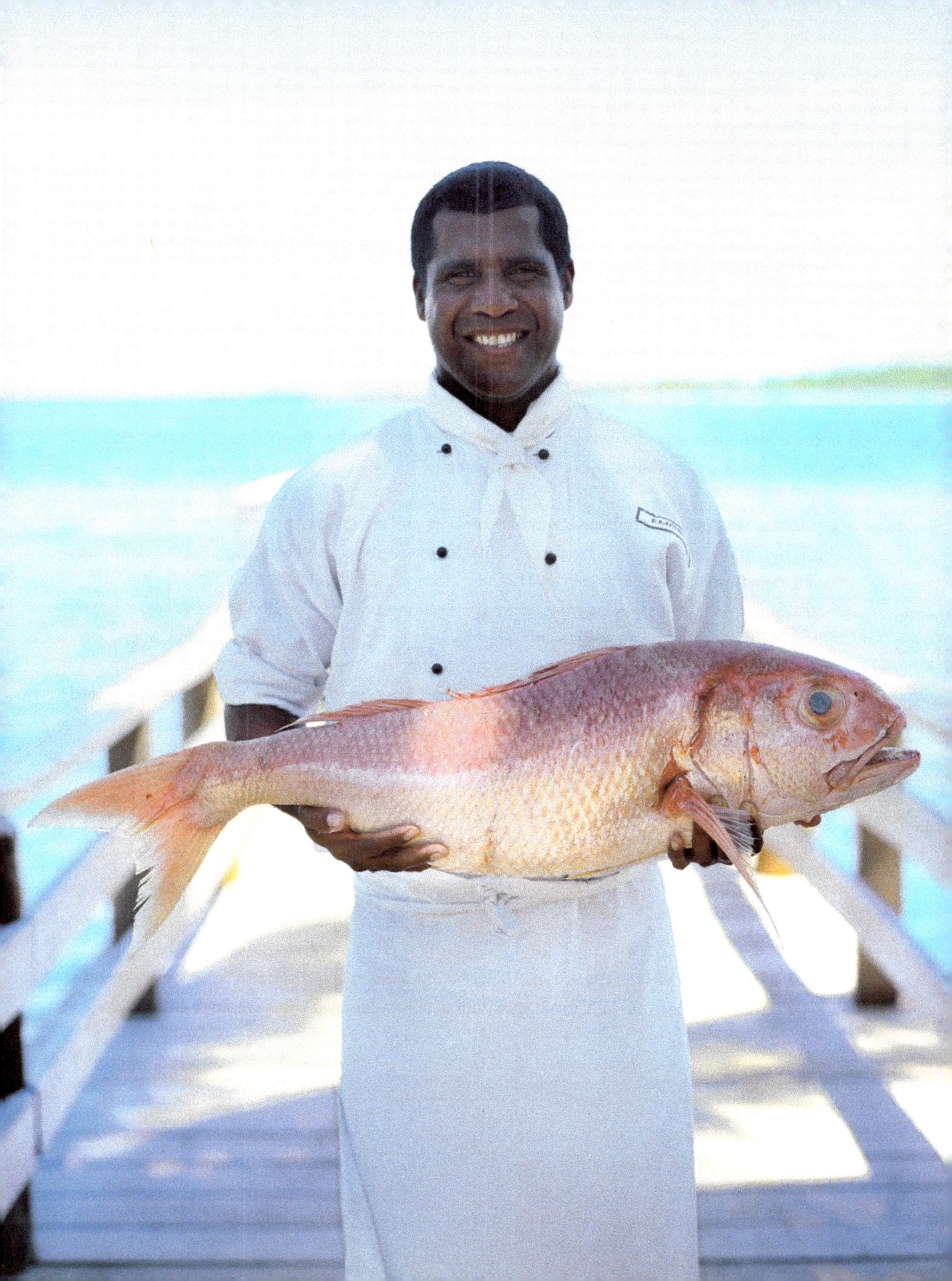

Juices

There is a lot of information out there about quitting sugar - but you don't need to be afraid of fruit, especially whole, fresh fruit. You'll never consume too much fructose if you're eating the entire fruit (imagine eating fi ve oranges at once!).

However, if you're planning on juicing, it's important to opt for plenty of vegetables such as celery, carrots, beetroot, spinach and broccoli, then sweeten with piece of fruit. Avoid fruit-only or packaged juices as they're high in sugar and won't fi ll you up.

Juices offer a great way to increase raw food intake and also a fun alternative to get your kids to eat their fruit and vegetables if you have fussy eaters.

Sometimes you just need to have some extra energy and a feeling of a fresh start.
This is one of my favourite juices to make to feel 'detoxed', energised and ready for the day ahead. Balancing a fresh squeeze with kale and beetroot brings the sugar levels down and creates a better GI, rather than just juicing fruits and high sugar ingredients. You don't have to avoid sugar altogether but including vegetables and other alkaline components is an ideal combination.
I always add some essential greens such as Kale, Spinach or even broccoli to my juices to up my antioxidant intake and increase the nutritional value. Other good additions are ginger and grated coconut... But here's today's JUICE OF THE DAY!

What's in it:
Beetroot
Apple
Carrot
Kale
Lime

Juicing is a fantastic way to increase your inner health, energy levels and raw food intake. It's also a fun alternative to get your kids to eat their fruit and vegetables if you have fussy eaters.

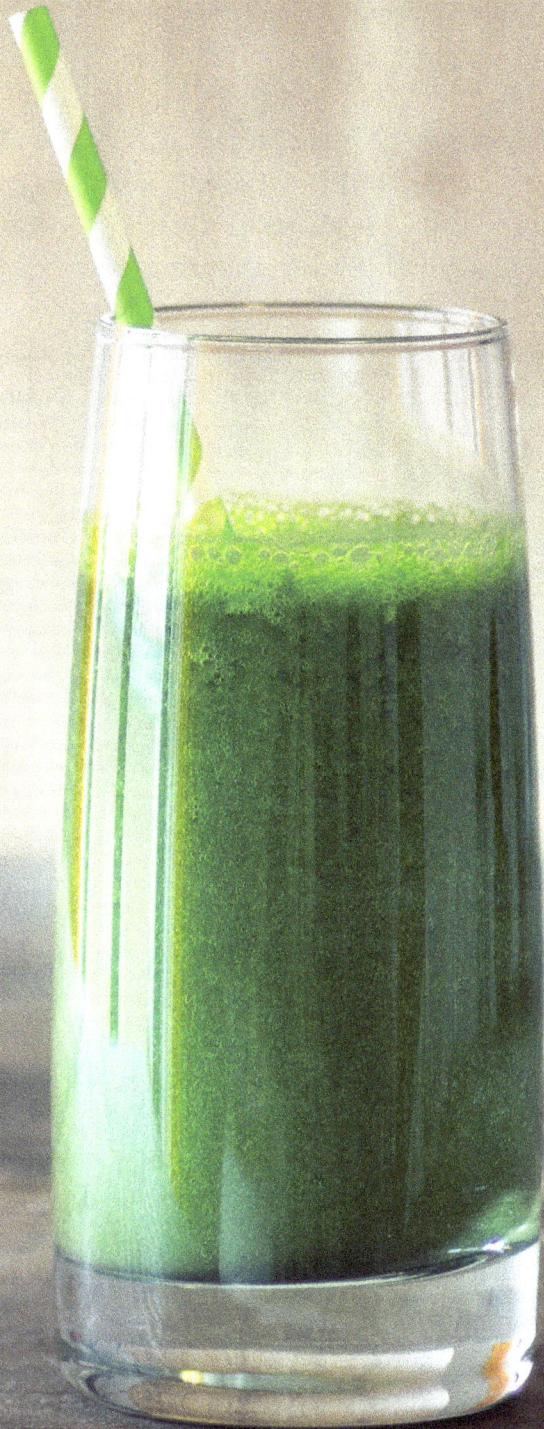

Breakfast

Breakfast is the key meal to kick-start your metabolism and ensure you're set for the day ahead. Most often misunderstood and misquoted, metabolism simply refers to the body breaking down foods into smaller molecules to allow absorption, and then reassembling them to form desired compounds.

It's a process that occurs throughout the body at all times but is highest when the body has food to break down or needs to build muscle or repair tissue after exercise. Our muscles burn calories even when we're sleeping, so ensuring we're maintaining lean muscle tissue through diet and exercise will in turn help us lose weight when we're just sitting around.

Eating a healthy breakfast is essential to provide nutritional support for your day and can help over-eating later on. Once again keep an eye on your portion sizes, making sure you include a source of protein and fibre.

Bircher Muesli

Ingredients:
1-2 cup Bircher muesli (I use Brookfarm Bircher, but you can use your own creation)
1/4 cup chopped almonds, sunflower seeds or hazelnuts
1/2 cup frozen or fresh blueberries
1/2 cup almond milk
1-2 tablespoons chia seeds
1 grated green apple, skin on

Preparation:
Mix the muesli with your almond milk, grated apple, nuts, blueberries and chia seeds. Leave in the fridge, covered, to soak overnight (or at least one hour). To serve, stir then add a splash of almond milk and sprinkle extra blueberries on top.

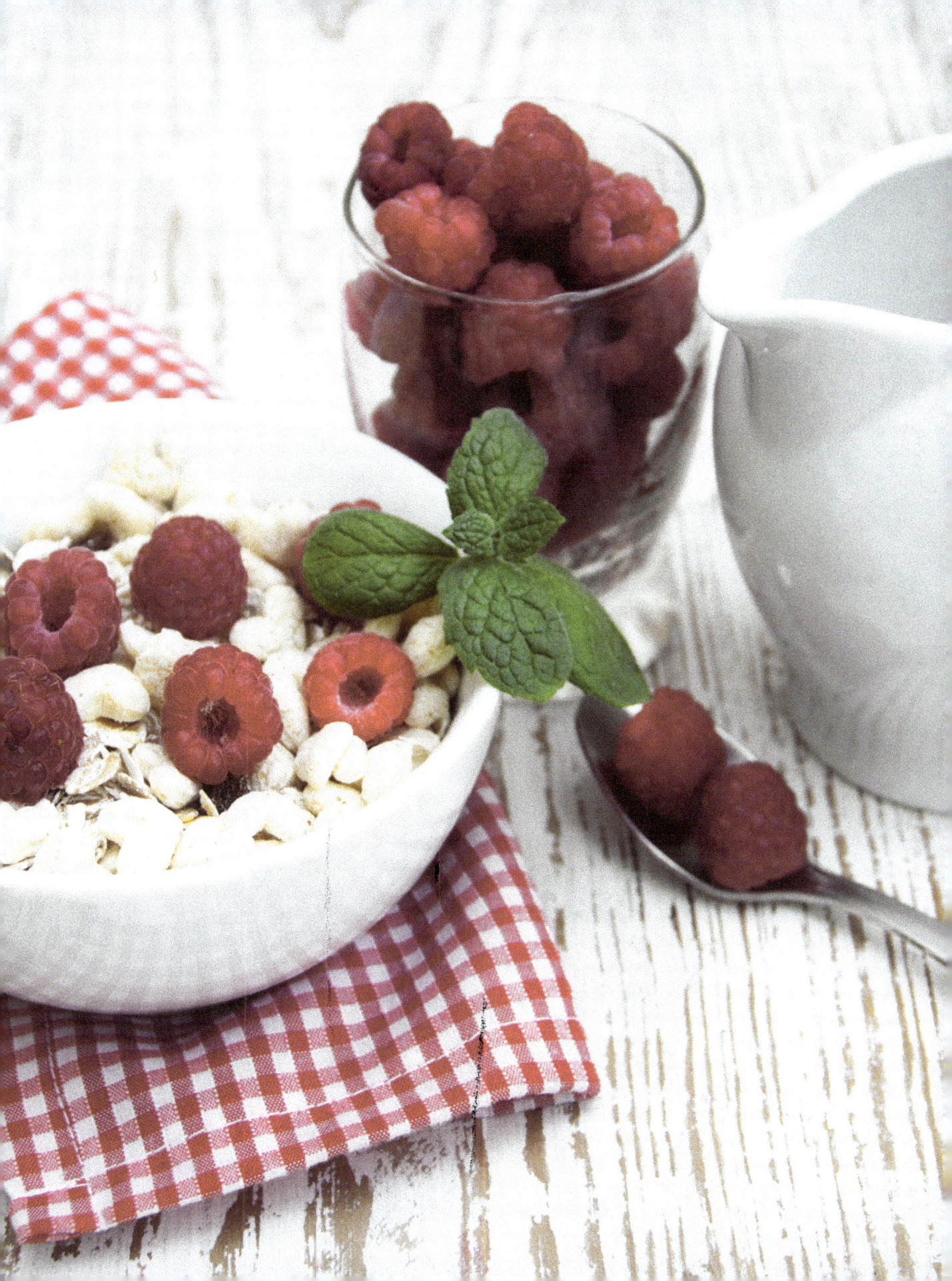

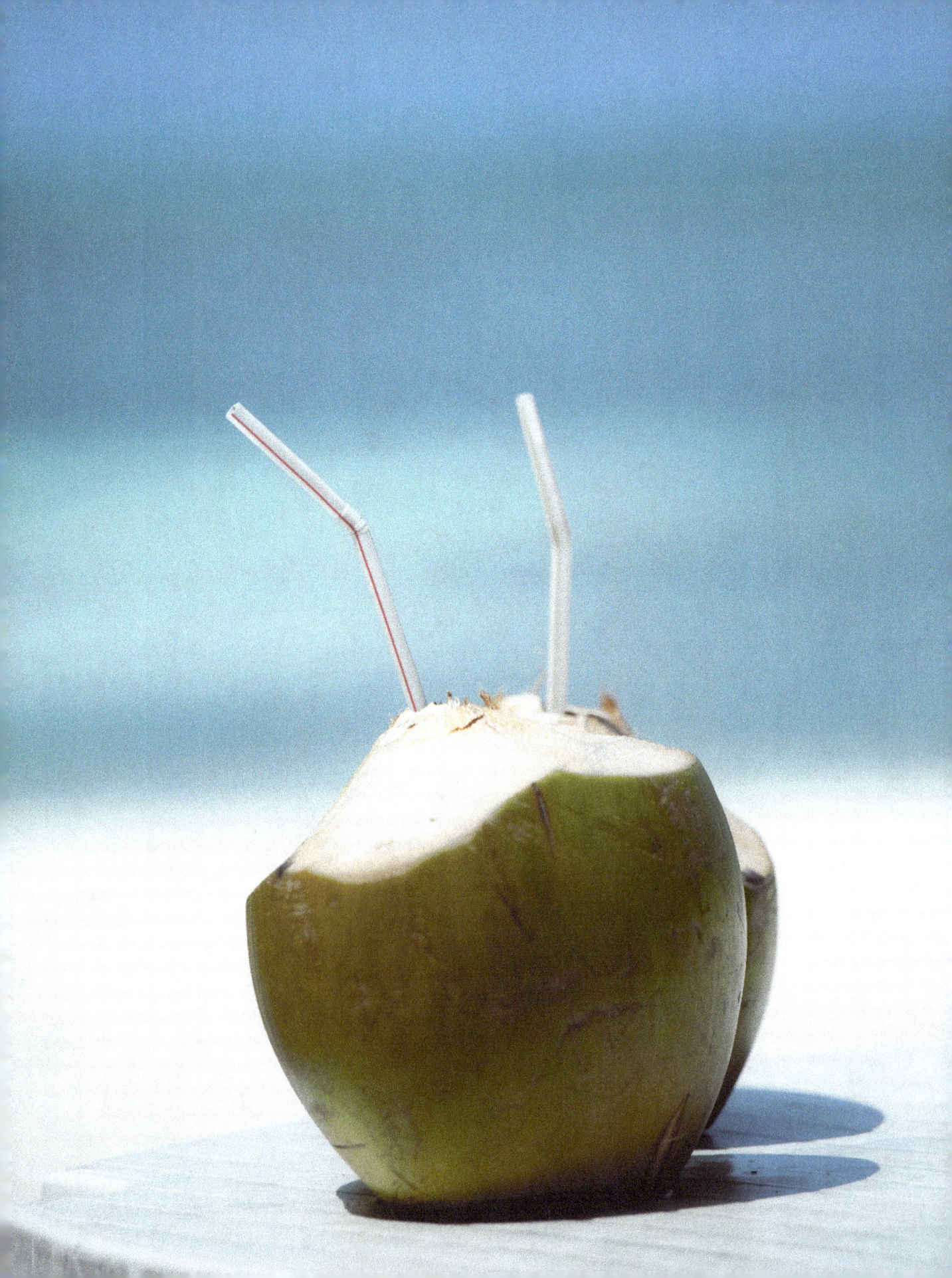

Oh My Omelette!

My 'emergency omelette' is a guaranteed winner! And it's perfectly okay to eat breakfast for dinner – provided you know how to make a healthy breakfast!

Ingredients:

3 lightly whisked eggs (3 whites, 2 yolks)
Fresh and frozen vegetables of your choice
Chopped fresh herbs, if available
1 tablespoon cheese (goat cheese is my pick)
1/2 tablespoon macadamia oil, or other oil suitable for frying

Preparation:

Put the veggies and oil into a non-stick pan on medium heat. Cook for five minutes or until the onion is just clear, then toss in your egg mixture. Throw in some cheese and chopped herbs. Cook gently then fold one side over to make an omelette. Slide out of pan on to your plate and add chopped cucumber, avocado and rocket on top for an extra special breakfast meal.

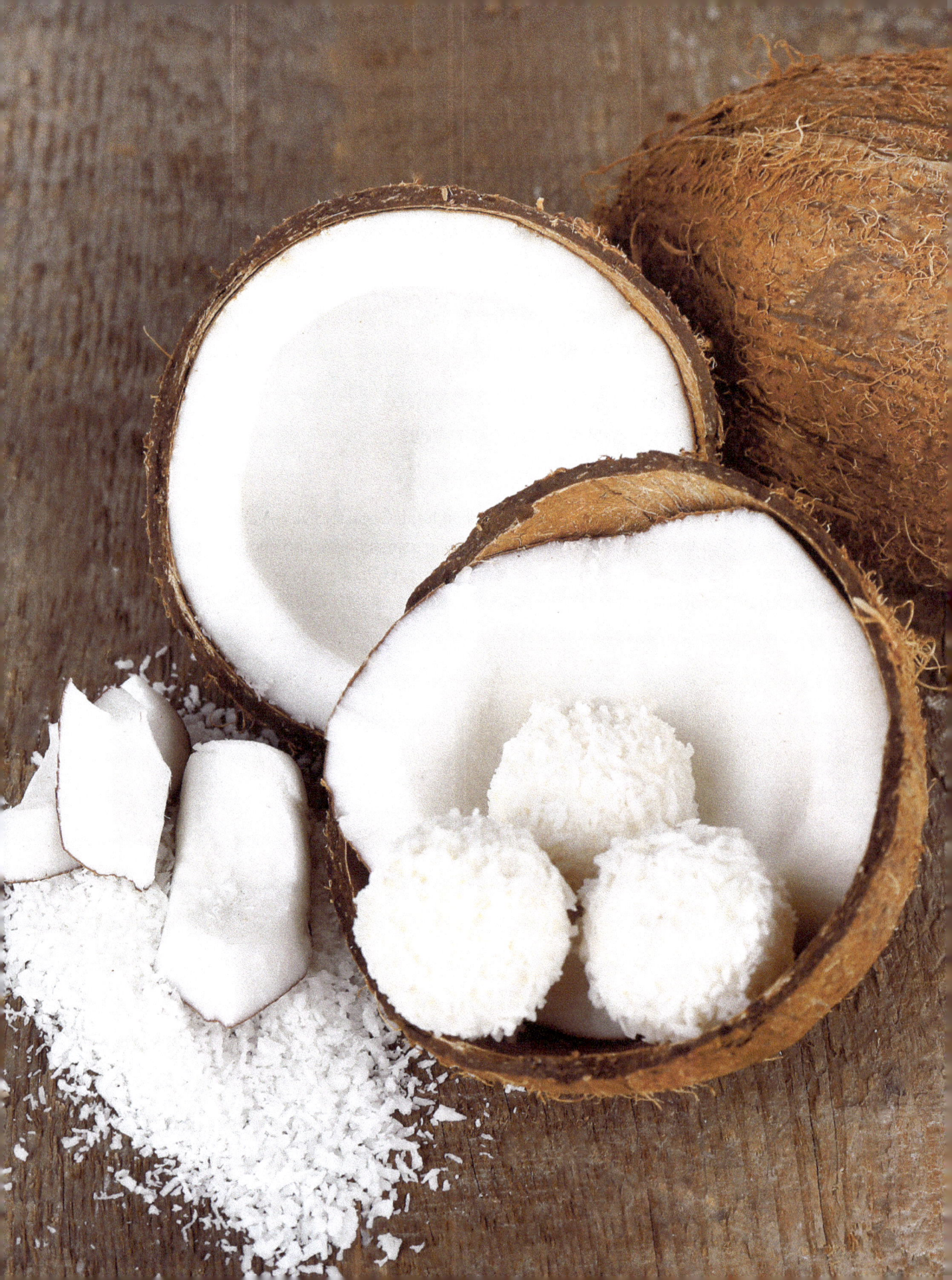

Morning munchies

Why all this talk of protein and regular small snacks throughout the day?
It's because it assists with muscle repair (maintaining lean muscle mass) and limits cravings by giving you a more satisfied feeling, partly due to its regulation of blood glucose levels.

It's essential for lasting weight loss, sustained energy and overall health! The goal when preparing snacks is to create a mini-meal with sustainable, healthy carbs and quality protein in every bite.

Bliss balls

Ingredients:

1 cup pitted or fresh dates
1/4 cup raw almonds
1 cup walnuts
5 pitted prunes
2 scoops of natural protein powder
1 chopped protein bar (optional)
Shredded coconut
2 tbs chia seeds
Lime zest

Nikki's tip:
It's a good idea to soak the nuts and dates overnight to make them easier to blend – or even 15 minutes in hot water.

Preparation:

Place all the ingredients in a food processor and blend until smooth. Add a touch of filtered water and some squeezed lime juice until you get the consistency right. It should be sticky and not too dry, making it easy to roll into a ball. Scoop a tablespoon out at a time, roll into a ball then roll in either sesame seeds or shredded coconut. Place in fridge or freezer and enjoy!

Smoothies

Smoothies and blended greens are an excellent way to enjoy a delicious drink that satisfies hunger and can offer fantastic nutrition. It's great to make them at home where you can control exactly what goes in.

If you're out and about, be mindful of ingredients as restaurants will choose flavour over health. Make sure whatever you order is free from sweetened yoghurt, ice cream, sugary syrups, artificial sweeteners and packaged juices.

Choose smoothies based on coconut water or nut milks with lots of fruit and vegetables, rather than those based on cow's milk or fruit juice. Then make sure you're including a source of protein, whether that's a powder or nuts/seeds.

Nikki's tip:
Think of smoothies
as a small meal or snack and
remember, they will be higher
in energy (calories) than
juices, so drink sparingly.

Apple Spinach and Mint Juice

(juice all the below ingredients and top with some crushed ice and mint leaves)

5 green apples
4 celery stalks
100g baby spinach leaves
2 cups mint leaves
1 lime, peeled

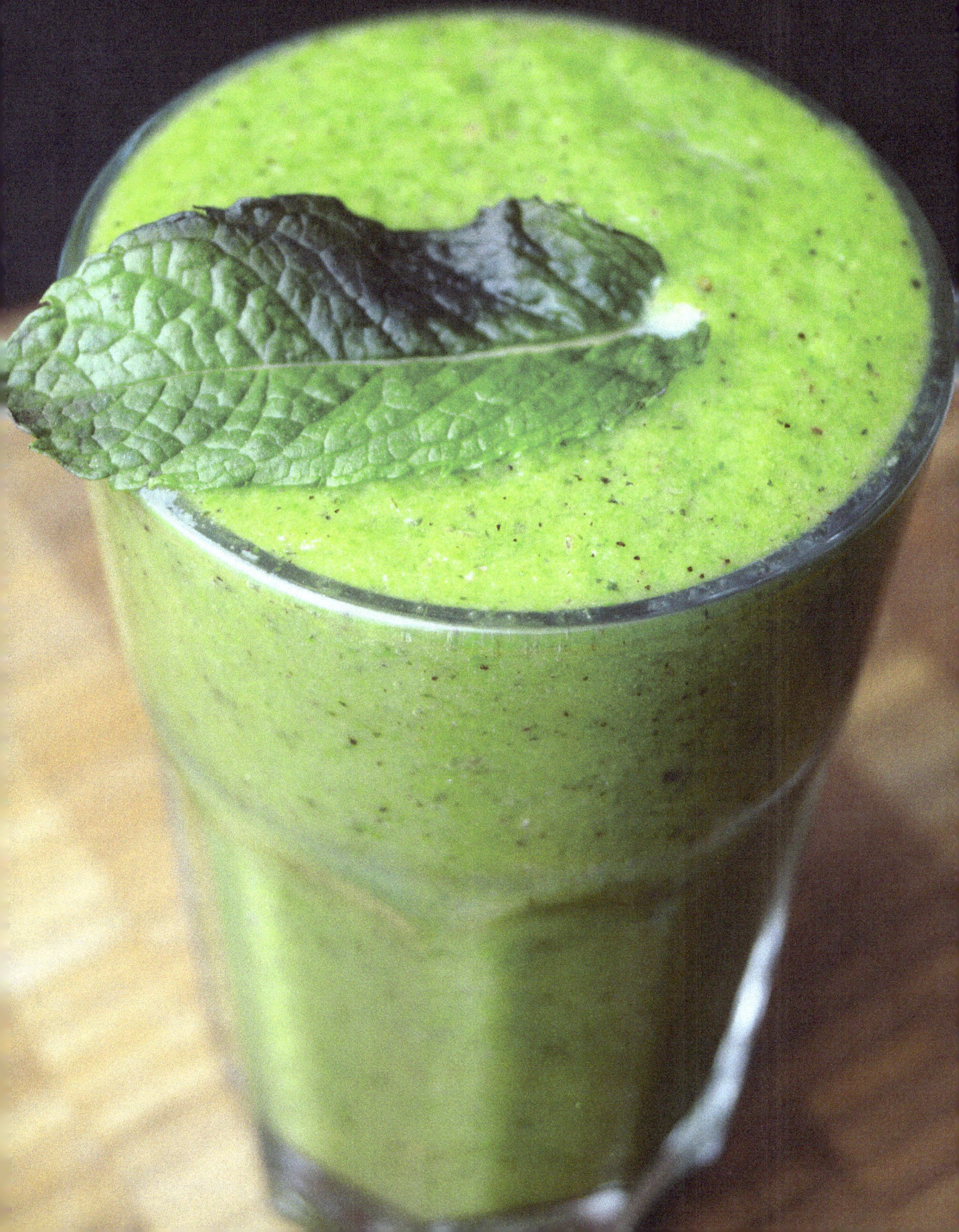

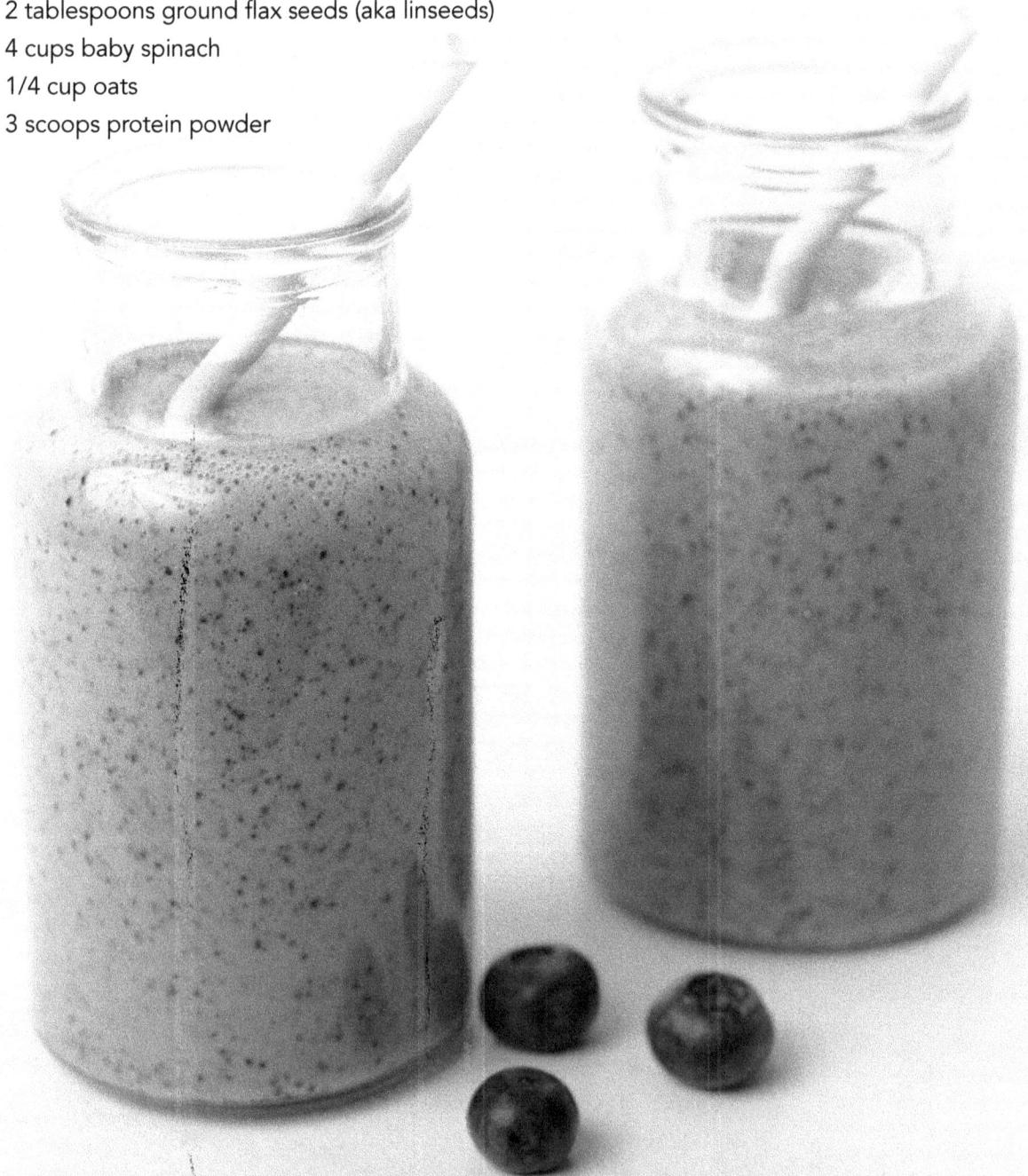

Blueberry dream

Ingredients:

1 cup fresh or frozen blueberries

1 banana, fresh or frozen

2 cups coconut water, almond or rice milk

1/2 avocado

4 dates (make sure you remove the pits!)

2 tablespoons ground flax seeds (aka linseeds)

4 cups baby spinach

1/4 cup oats

3 scoops protein powder

Super smoothie

Ingredients:

2 scoops of gluten-free Body Science Naturals protein powder (or equivalent)

1 Frozen banana

1/2 frozen mango

1 fresh or frozen kiwifruit

1/2 cup blueberries, fresh or frozen

1/2 avocado

2 cups coconut water, almond milk or filtered water

1-2 teaspoons Maca powder

1-2 tablespoons chia seeds

1 cup spinach

Ice

Add all ingredients to the blender and whizz. Pop any extra smoothie in a jar with a lid in the fridge for later in the day. Each recipe Serves 2.

The Fighting Fit Smoothie

Ingredients:

1/3 cup walnuts or cashews

1 generous handful baby spinach

1/2 cup blueberries, frozen or fresh

1 banana, frozen or fresh

1 cup non-dairy milk (soy, almond, coconut) or coconut water

1 serve of protein powder (optional)

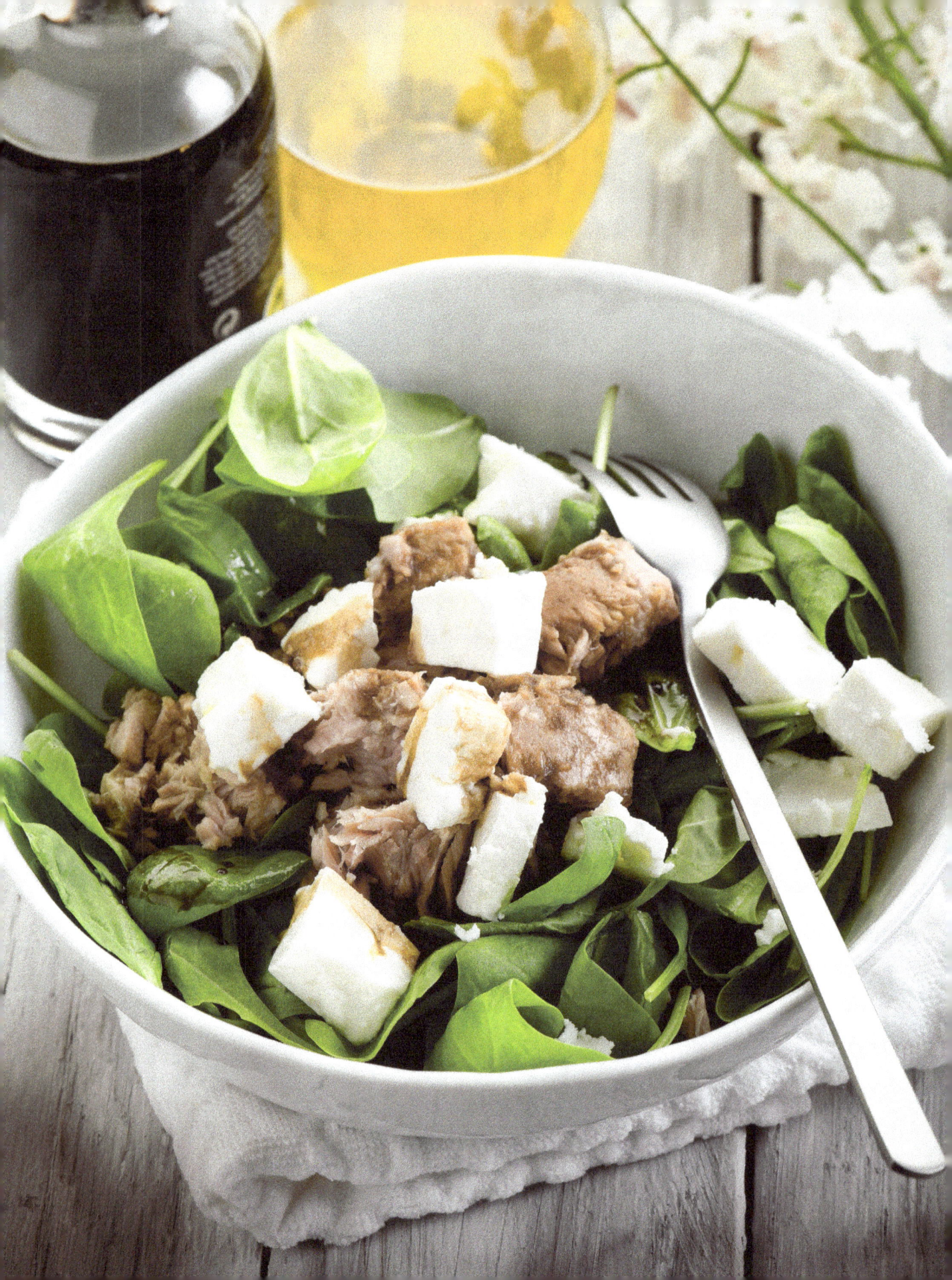

Lunch

Lunch is another fantastic opportunity to incorporate more fresh foods, help prevent afternoon snacking and that 3pm fuzziness.

Again, we're looking for a balanced meal containing a good amount of protein and fibre to keep you full throughout the afternoon. I know lunch can be tricky as work and life can get in the way, so being prepared is essential.

Pack leftovers, create something fresh or select smart restaurant items that will help you maintain a stable blood glucose level, keeping your body and brain firing until dinner.

Wok's Up!

Ingredients:
Fresh herbs
Mixed vegetables – your choice
Brown rice
Leftover meat or tofu

Preparation:
This dish is designed to pep up your metabolism and use whatever may be in your fridge. Throw in as many fresh herbs and vegetables as you can, as well as leftover or pre-cooked brown rice and tofu or lean organic meat and toss it around with vigour. Serve with a drizzle with lime juice and black pepper. If you like it hot, add some chopped chillies.

Eggs with homemade pesto and avocado on toasted sourdough

Ingredients:

2 eggs

1 slice of wholemeal sourdough or gluten free bread - or substitute this for a thin home baked and toasted pita bread

5 asparagus shoots

1 large clove of garlic

2 teaspoons macadamia or olive oil

1/2 lemon

Black pepper

Homemade pesto - pine nuts, parsley, pepper, walnuts - place all into a food processor and blend till smooth and creamy

1 avocado sliced

Preparation:

Place eggs in a saucepan and cover with cold water. Cover and bring to the boil over high heat. Add eggs and reduce heat to medium, then simmer gently for three minutes. Drain and rinse in cold water before carefully peeling. Meanwhile, heat oil in pan and gently fry crushed garlic until soft. Add asparagus shoots, and toss for another minute with a squeeze of lemon and black pepper. Serve asparagus on toast with eggs on top. Add avocado on top of the eggs and asparagus.

Afternoon snacks

The afternoon can be a risky time when you're trying to eat healthily and avoid tempting treats. It's a time when being prepared is especially important to help you say no to the cookie jar.

Having nutritious snacks available is the key to success. Make sure you always have the following on hand; you can prepare these in one afternoon on the weekend, then store them in handy snack-sized bags to grab and go during the week:

Raw nuts and sultanas
Veggie sticks (celery, cucumber, carrot etc) served with hummus
Fruit and natural yoghurt
Protein shakes will make life easier

Fit tip:
Avoid the caffeine hit and try having a green tea or simply water. This can help refresh your mind and also fill you up.

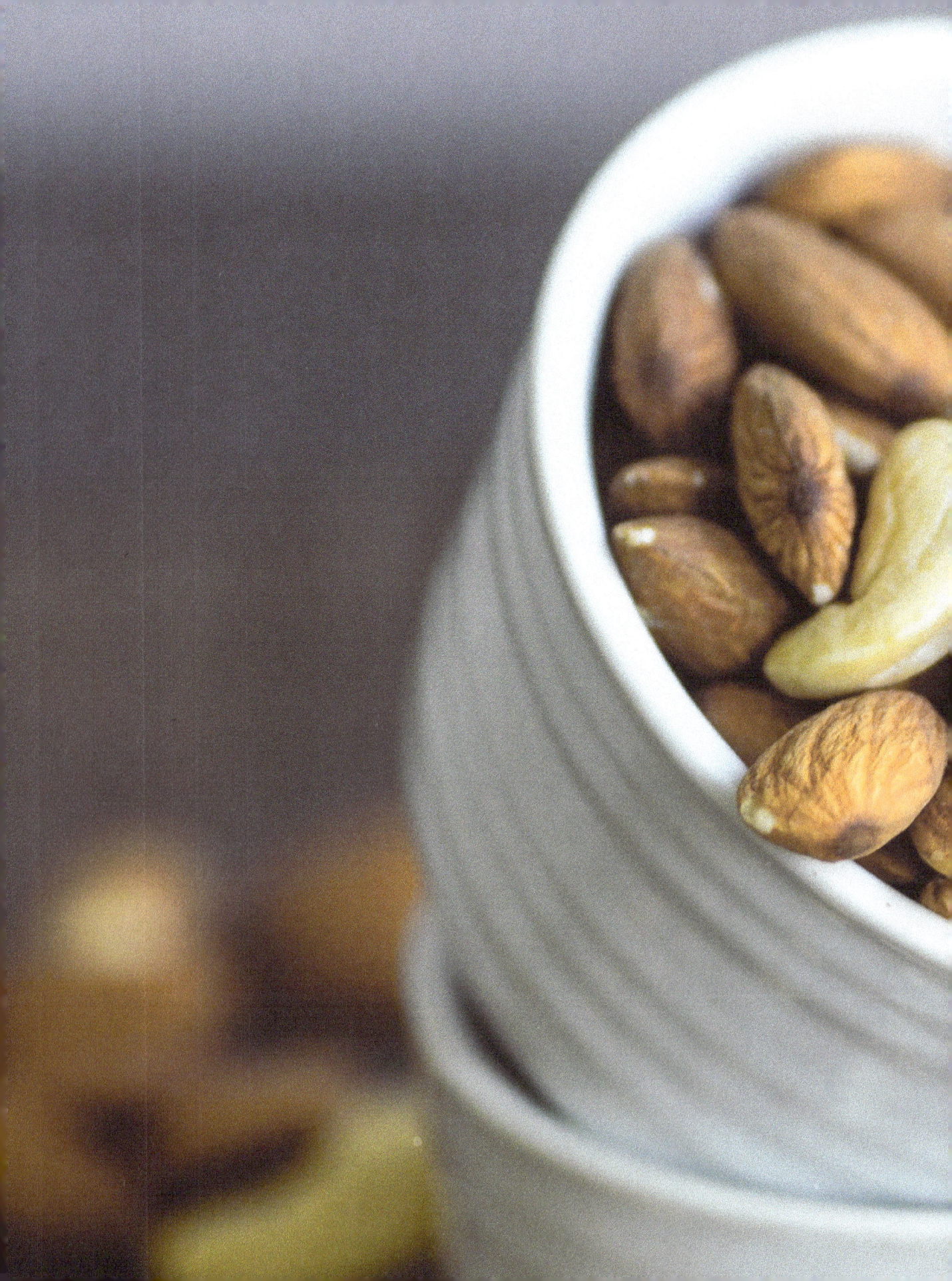

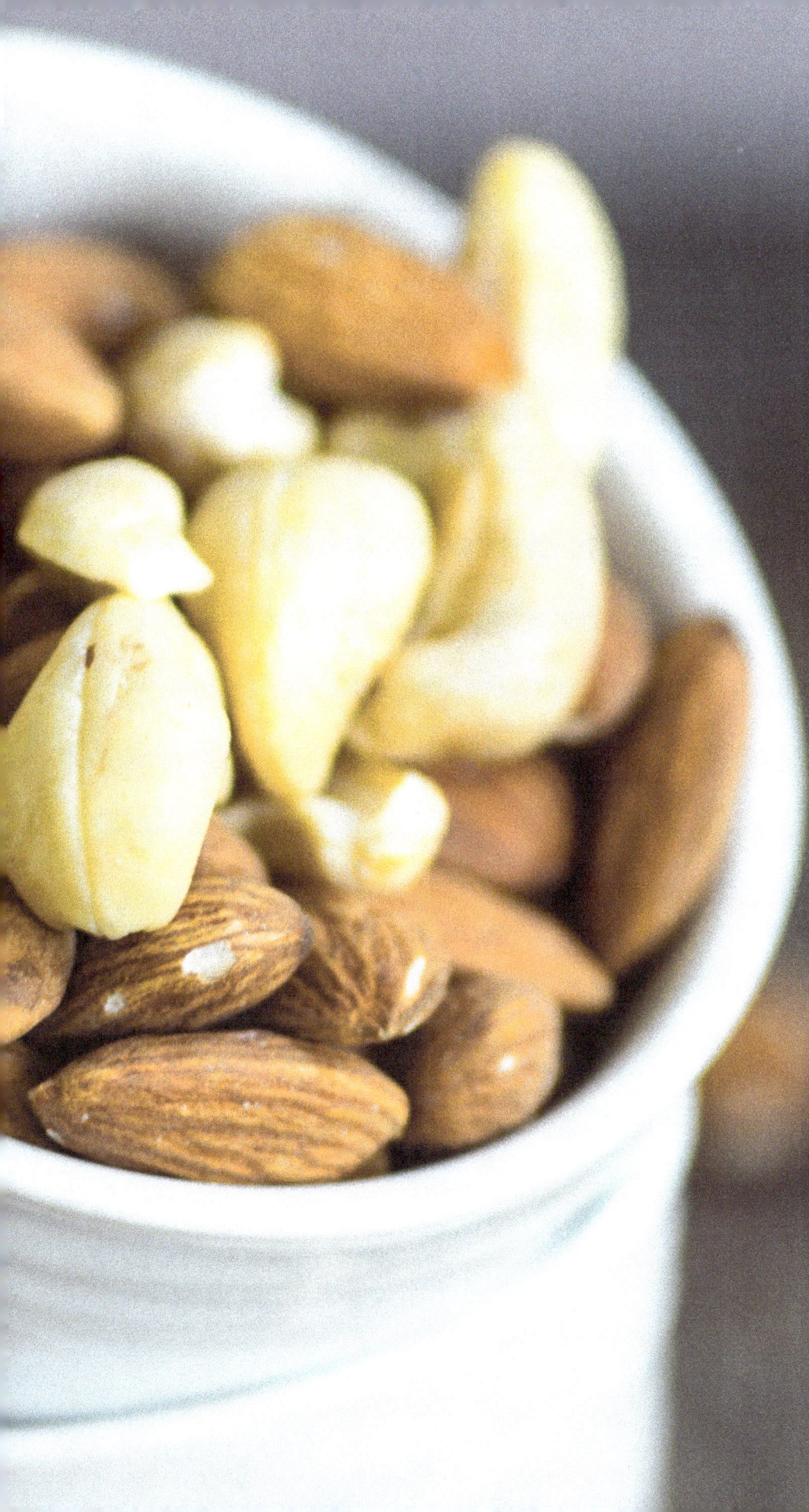

Dinner

Salads are a great base for your main meal of the day. But, if you're like me and you feel like you're on the go all the time, then you may find getting access to real, fresh greens and crunchy raw ingredients can be a little bit limiting.

Keeping your freezer well-stocked with vegetables and your pantry loaded with tinned legumes can provide some fantastic last-minute options. Making extra for the next day's lunch will also save you time and money later on and is one of those healthy habits worth cultivating.

Rocket, mango and goats cheese salad

Ingredients:
Rocket Mango Carrots Capsicum

Hard goat cheese

Walnuts

Macadamia oil (try the Brookfarm chilli infused macadamia oil)

Bean sprouts

Roma tomatoes

Cracked pepper

Grilled tofu, organic beef or chicken, or grilled salmon for on top of your salad.

Preparation:
Rinse and dry off any fresh ingredients, then mix all ingredients (except mango) in a bowl. Serve onto a plate and place mango slices on top, along with any protein choice and cracked pepper.

NOTE

Seared Salmon with rocket salad

Ingredients:

1 fillet of fish for each person

2 cups rocket per person

1 pear per person

Macadamia or cold pressed olive oil

Sea salt

1-2 limes

1/2 cup chopped walnuts

Wash and pat your salmon dry, adding a light coat of salt on the skin side. Set aside, ready to fry. Prepare your rocket salad by placing all ingredients straight into a serving bowl: wash and rinse the rocket, thinly slice your pear, drizzle with lime juice, macadamia or cold pressed olive oil, salt and toss around with some chopped walnuts. Heat a non-stick pan to medium and add one tablespoon of macadamia oil. Bring to the heat and add the salmon, skin-side first. Cook almost to your liking, ensuring the skin becomes nice and crispy, then finish cooking on the other side.

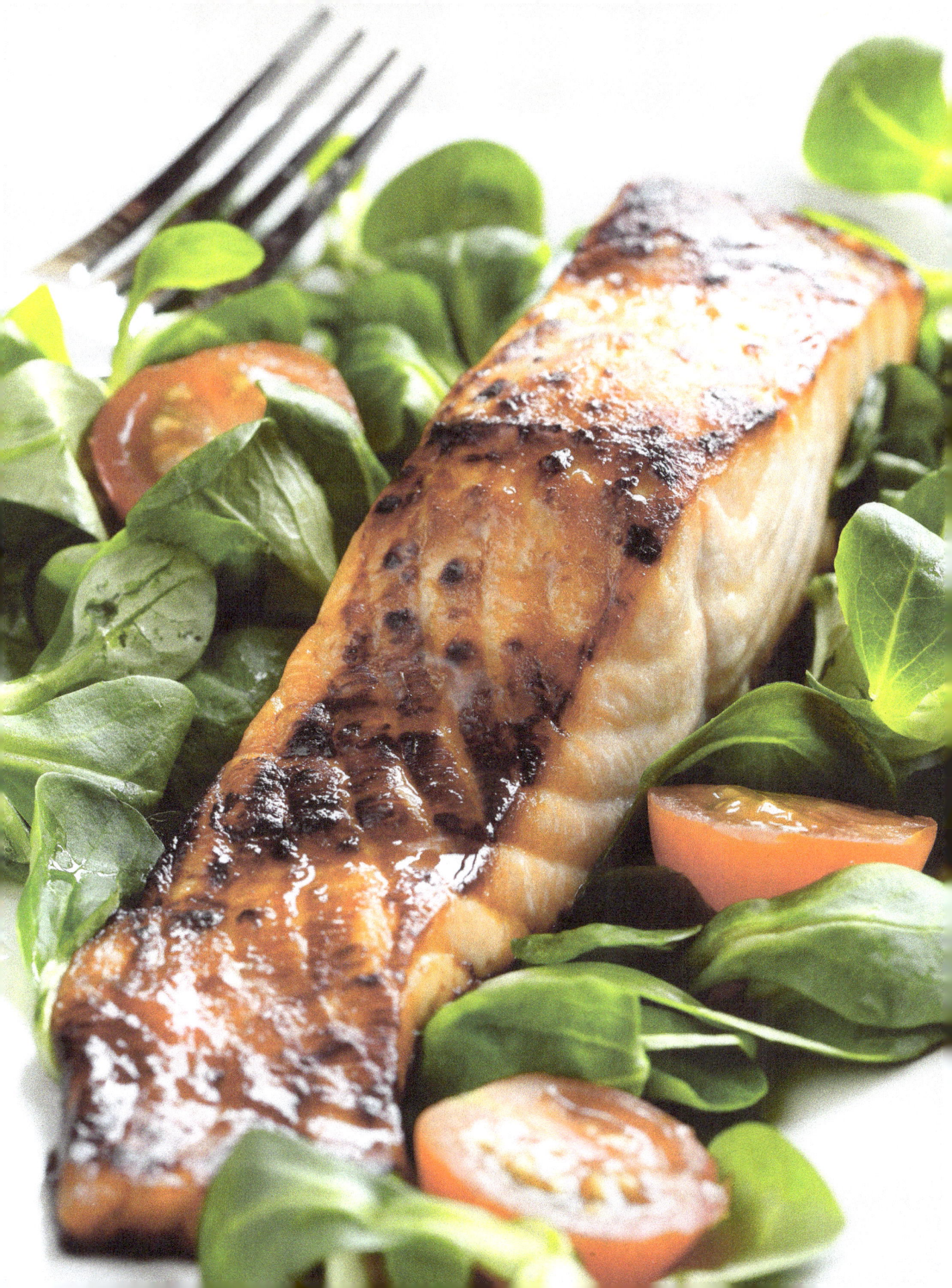

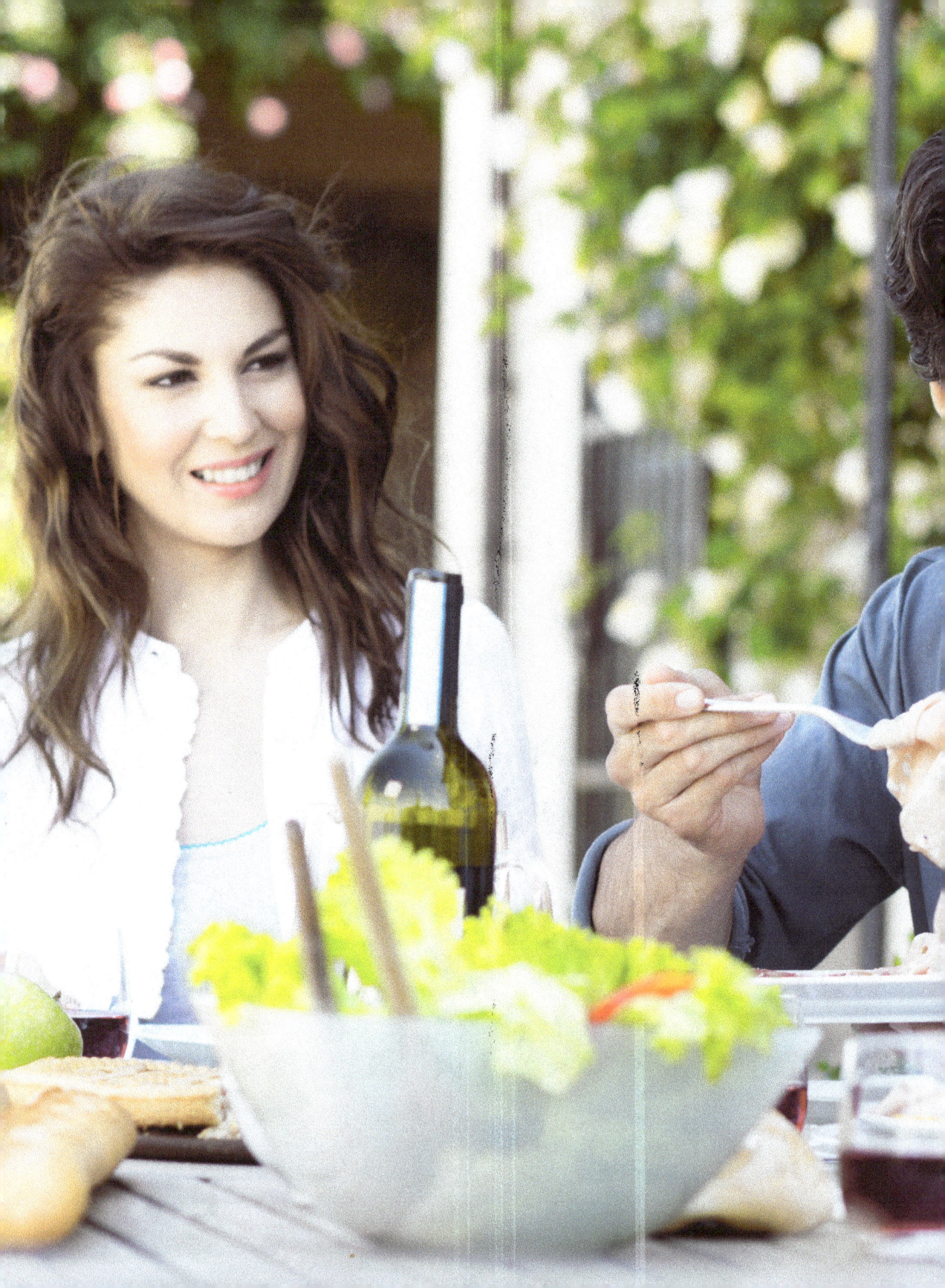

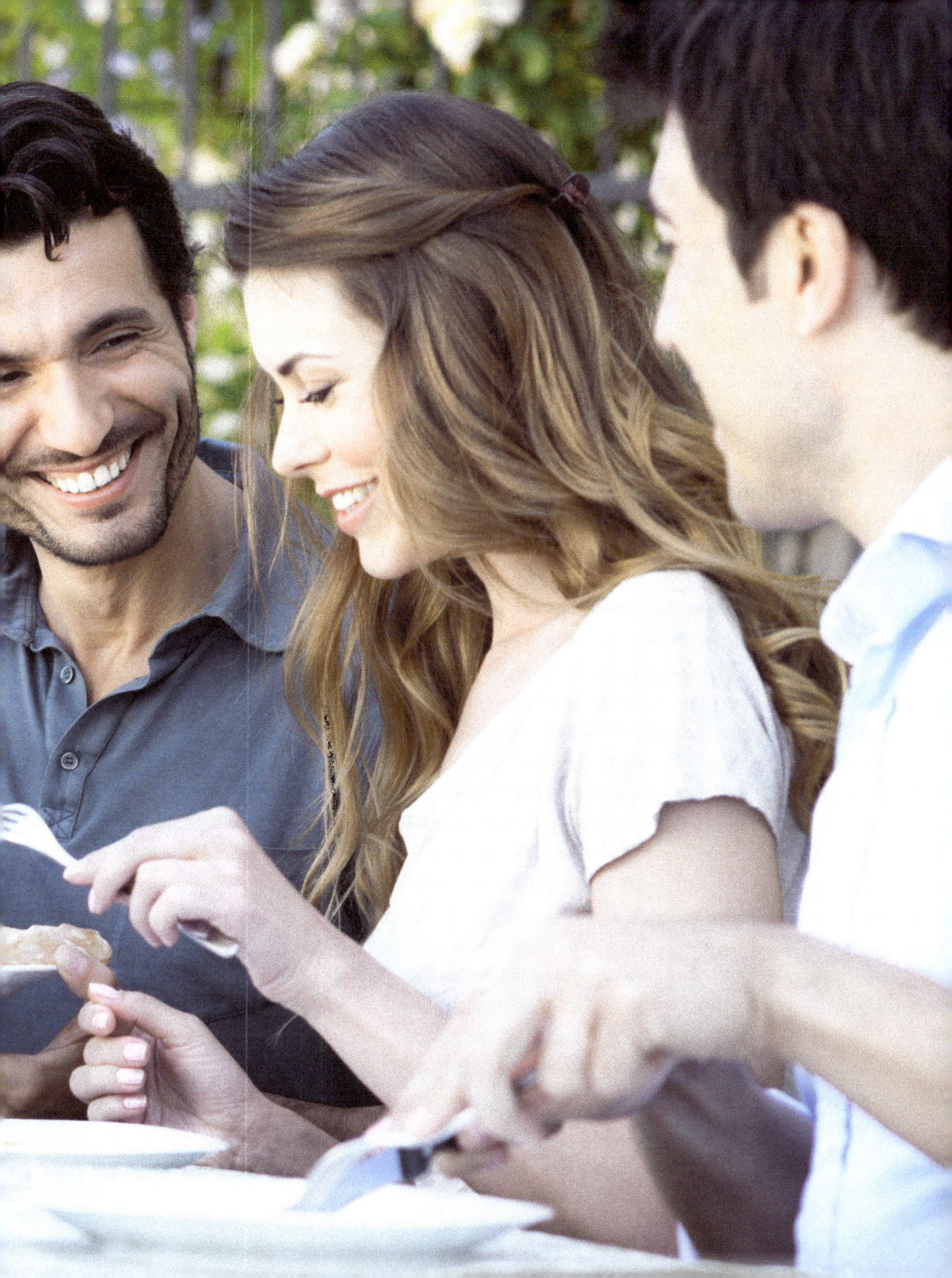

Evening munchies

If you have enough protein in each meal you should not be craving sugary desserts, but if you genuinely hungry, you may want a little something after your evening meal.

I use this time to have a light protein-rich and potassium-packed snack to aid muscle recovery over night and replenish minerals while sleeping.

Also remember to think about ensuring your main meal and each snack is abundant with natural colour for increased vitamin and antioxidant qualities. The more natural colour a dish has the better it is for you.

After dinner snack ideas:

6 pitted organic prunes

1/2 serve of natural protein powder with water and ice

2-3 Rye, gluten free or rice crackers with natural nut butter

Frozen banana with Maca powder in the blender (it makes a mousse-like dessert!)

Celery sticks or carrot with hummus

Nikki's tip:
Have some magnesium powder in the evenings if you have a busy schedule and are getting back into training, as this can help regulate and repair your system, and decrease restless legs and cramps.

★

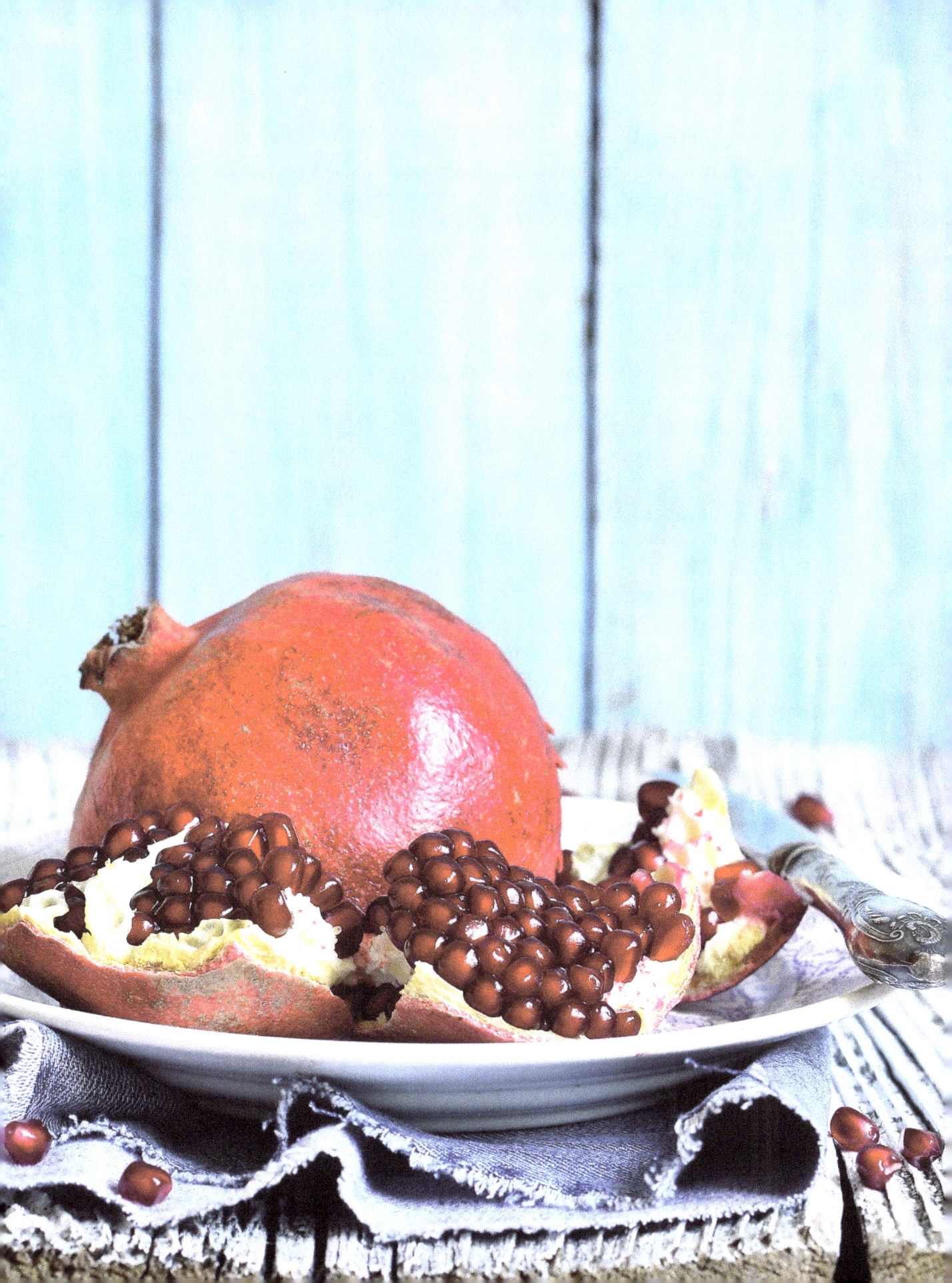

Tips when dining out

If, for 80% of the time, you keep up with your healthy living routine, the odd unhealthy meal here and there is not going to ruin it all. The key is to not feel like you've let yourself down and subsequently let all your hard work go out the window!

Enjoy being in the moment, knowing you look after yourself and you can't control everything. Here are some tips for making healthy choices when you're dining out or at someone else's house:
- ★ Drink plenty of water before you order.
- ★ If you want to have an alcoholic drink, opt for vodka lime and soda.
- ★ Avoid white wines and beers.
- ★ Skip the breads and tempting appetisers.
- ★ Look for words such as 'poached', 'steamed', 'baked', 'boiled' or 'grilled' and avoid anything 'fried', 'braised', 'buttered', 'au gratin' or 'creamed'.
- ★ If you must order dessert, share it with your date; you only ever really enjoy the first couple of bites anyway.

Ordering at Restaurants

Italian - Swap creamy Italian pastas and risottos, thick-crust pizzas and lasagna for tomato based sauces, fish and seafood soups or even thin-crust pizzas, order extra salad, ask for olive oil only as a dressing and look for grilled or fresh ingredients.
Asian - Choose veggie based stir-frys with oyster sauce and rice paper rolls instead of spring rolls
Pub - Go for steamed or grilled fish with salad and choose nicoise salads over Caesar salads - always ask for the dressing on the side
Mexican - Choose chilli con carne, fajitas or tacos instead of Nachos, burritos and enchiladas - I always ask for extra guacamole, salads and choose the options that come with a hot plate so I can make my own fajitas.

Fit family tips

Involve your children in cooking on the weekends and get them excited about food by discovering a local farmers market.

Lead by example and talk about food and nutrition with a positive outlook - make good choices for yourself and let your children see the amazing options available to them by introducing them to a healthy attitude about food. Avoid using the word diet and a list of foods you 'can't have' but instead focus on a massive list of foods and snacks that are tasty and fun to have in the house.

Nikki's tip

Have a busy household? Write up a list of afternoon snacks or breakfast ideas and print this out, laminate it and place it on the fridge or inside of the pantry so your family members have a quick reference list of ideas for healthy snacks and breakfasts when they are in a hurry.

Staying healthy on the go

If you're on the road, travelling or simply busy, it pays to be prepared. Pack yourself snacks so you don't make poor or desperate decisions. Fill your office draw, handbag or car with healthy snacks and research healthy cafes or restaurants in the area.

The fact that our body enzymes cannot break it down ensures that fibre acts as a binding agent for toxins, escorting substances we don't need safely out of the body and avoiding fermentation, or nasty build-up in our bodies and disease.

Fibre is essential for a healthy digestive system and should not be overlooked in your daily diet. You need both forms of insoluble and soluble fibre for optimal health, hence the benefit of eating whole food, instead of their extracted and processed versions

Supplements and packaged foods are no substitute for fresh, whole foods, but if you're travelling you need to be prepared.

A healthy amount of natural dietary fibre per day can assist with:

★ Lowering cholesterol levels.

★ Minimising chronic inflammation and associated diseases.

★ Reducing the risk of bowel cancer and potentially other cancers.

★ Symptoms associated with Irritable Bowel Syndrome (IBS).

★ Diabetes and managing blood glucose levels.

★ Maintaining healthy gut bacteria.

Soluble fibre: Acts like a sponge when it's combined with water and absorbs toxins and waste, making them easier to extract from the body. Eg. fruits, vegetables, avocado, oat bran, barley, seed husks, flaxseed, psyllium, dried beans, lentils, peas, and organic natural soy milk and soy products.

PS: A WORD ON FIBRE DIETARY FIBRE IS FOUND IN THE INDIGESTIBLE PARTS OF PLANTS. IF IT'S IN THE INDIGESTIBLE PARTS OF PLANTS, I HEAR YOU ASK, THEN HOW CAN IT BE GOOD FOR US?

Insoluble fibre: Is found in the structural parts of plant cell walls and does not bind with water, but is essential in creating bulk and prevents constipation. Without efficient elimination of waste, your body won't run on its full potential. Eg. wheat bran, corn bran, rice bran, the skins of fruits and vegetables, nuts, seeds, dried beans and whole grain foods.

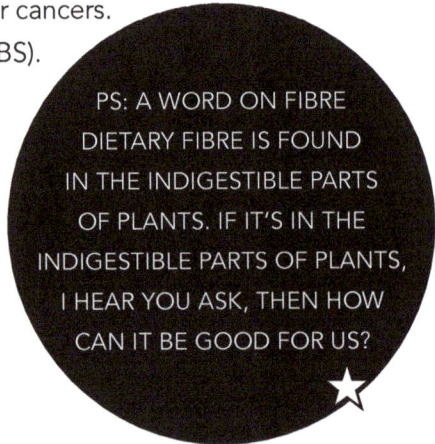

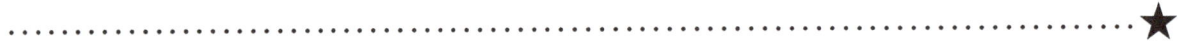

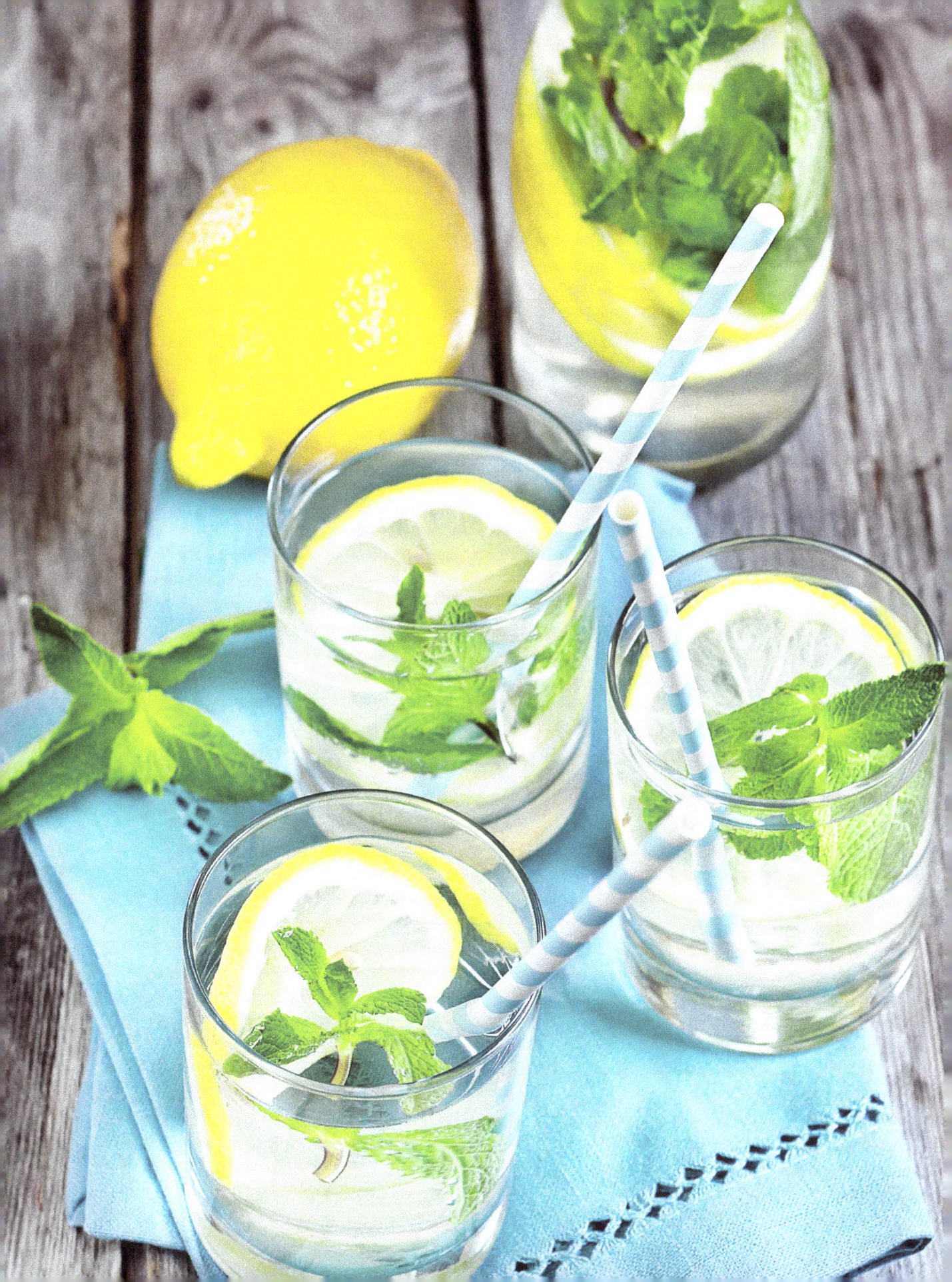

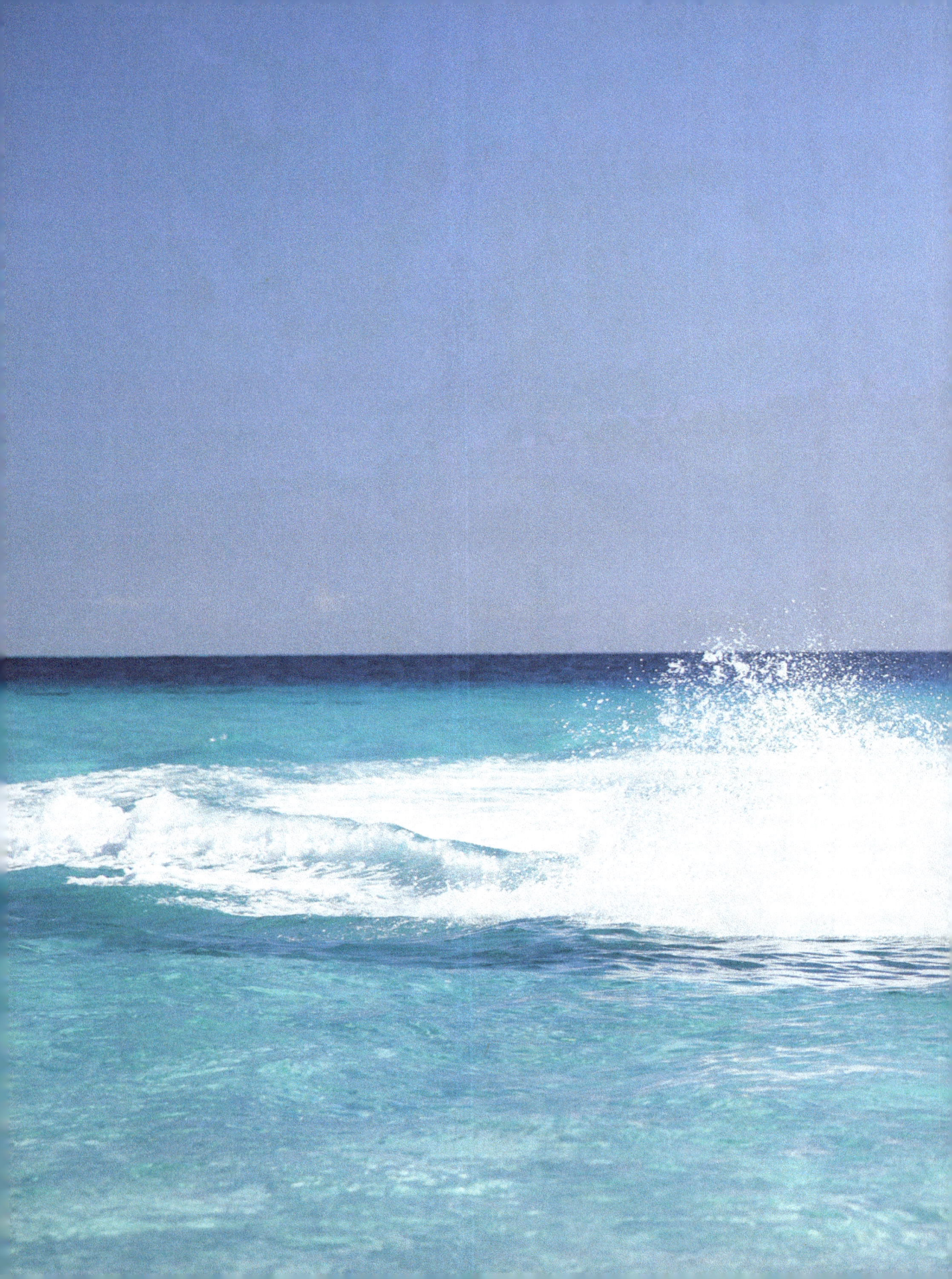

CHAPTER FOUR:
LIVING THE LIFE YOU LOVE

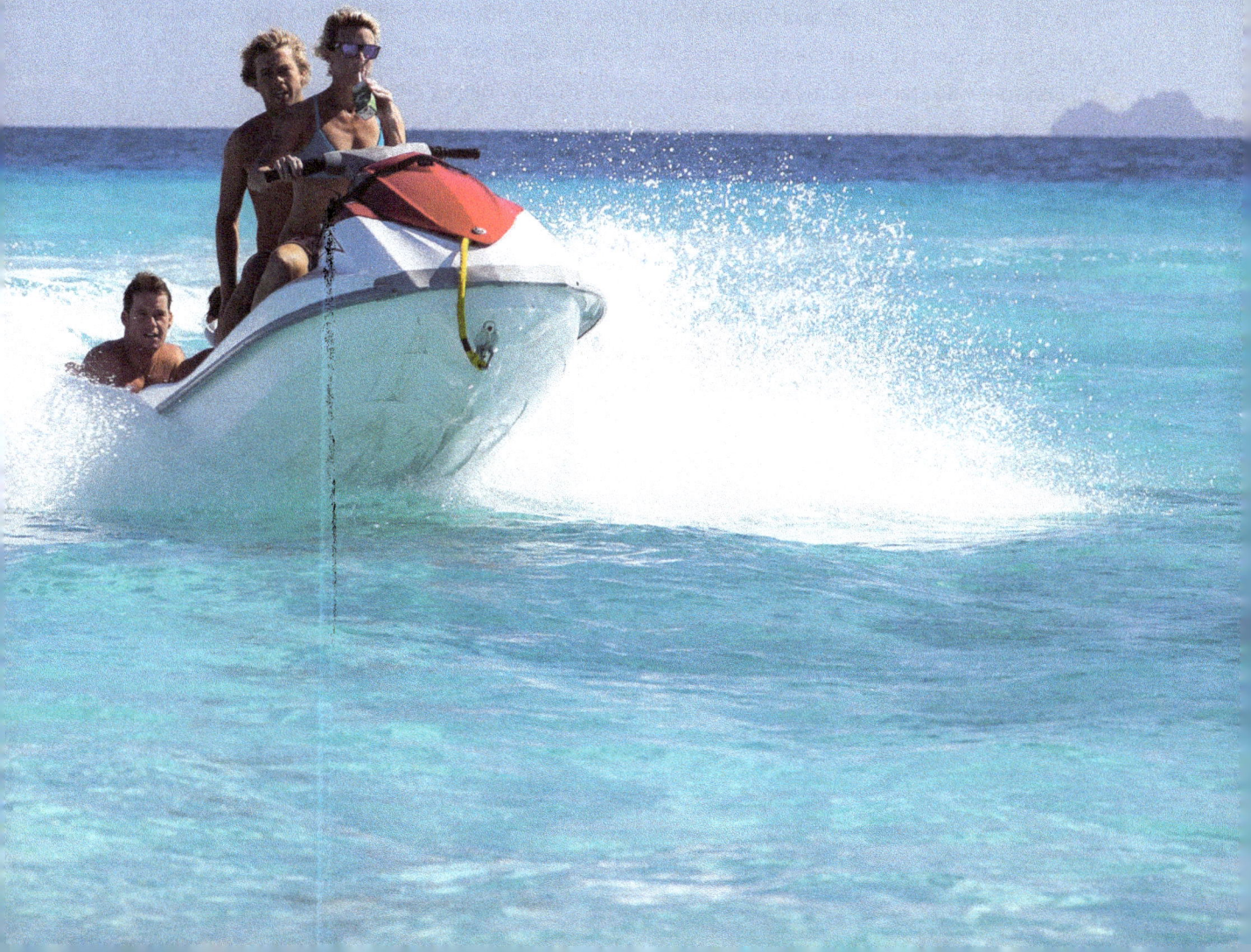

So you've made it this far.

By now, you've probably realised I'm a big believer that you create the life you want.

It is entirely your decision. Stay where you are or decide to move forward and open up your world: those are your choices. Life has no remote – you must get up and change it yourself and it's never to late to look and feel fantastic and refresh your goals.

If you truly want to be your personal best, then you're going to need to accept challenges in your life and say yes to opportunities as they present themselves. Even if, on a small-scale, you can do just one thing every seven days that is out of your comfort zone, you will be moving in the right direction of creating change and development.

Set yourself a challenge

Creating your own personal challenge is crucial for your sense of confi dence and accomplishment. Set a date, get your friends and family involved and write down something that you've always wanted to achieve. It could be swimming 100 laps of your local pool; running 10km without slowing to a walk; hiking somewhere as an adventure; or joining a charity fi tness event. Whatever it is, make sure it's fun and most importantly – commit yourself to reaching your goal at all costs!

I did this myself, when I recently competed in one of the top 10 adventure races in the world: The Mark Webber Tasmania Challenge. Our team had never been in an adventure race in our lives, had never been orienteering and all three of us came from completely different disciplines.

This was a challenge in every sense: mind, body and soul were about to be tested over fi ve gruelling days. Even though we were a team, we were all there for our own individual growth and sense of challenge.

Fit tip:
Look further afield and choose a goal that is bigger than normal and completely out of your comfort zone to aim towards. Make sure it truly excites you and is something you WANT to do; it will make the sense of accomplishment you feel afterwards that much more satisfying!

It might have hurt like heck and tested our physical limits, our patience and our navigation skills all at once – but we absolutely stuck to our guns, whatever it took. I am extremely proud of our team, our resilience, our open-minded approach and our sense of spirit that kept us laughing throughout those five days.

I also wholeheartedly believe that it is not until we're tested that we learn more about ourselves. We can take the new road and the chance to step up, be confronted and grow, or we stay with the path we know, shy away from something new and daunting, and maintain the status quo.

Do the little voices tell you…

"It's not possible"

"I'm not fit enough"

"I can't do that"

"I haven't trained"

"I'm not qualified"

"It s not my place to ask…"

Recognise these as they pop up and then push them away with a sense of conviction that you can do anything you put your mind to!

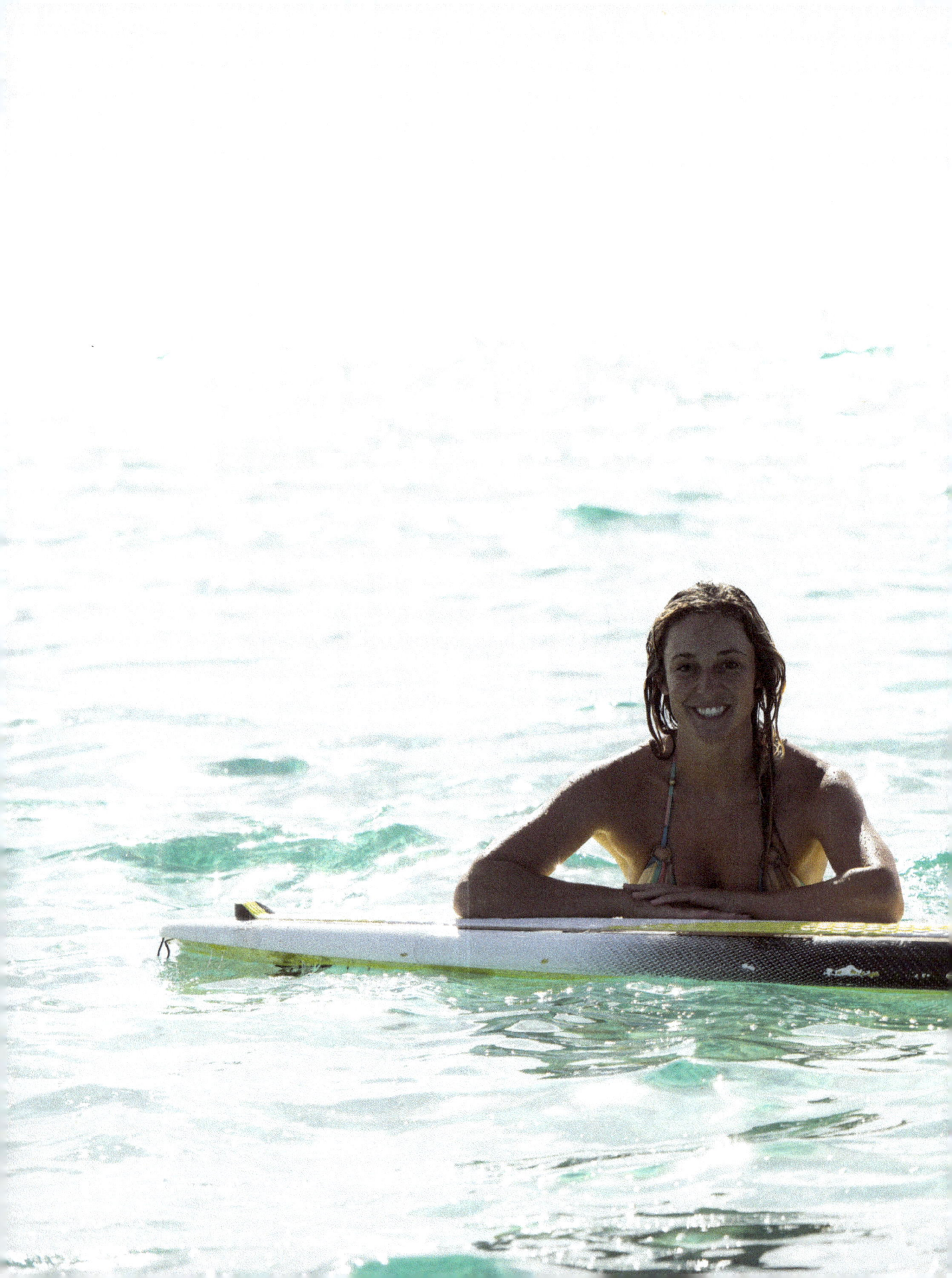

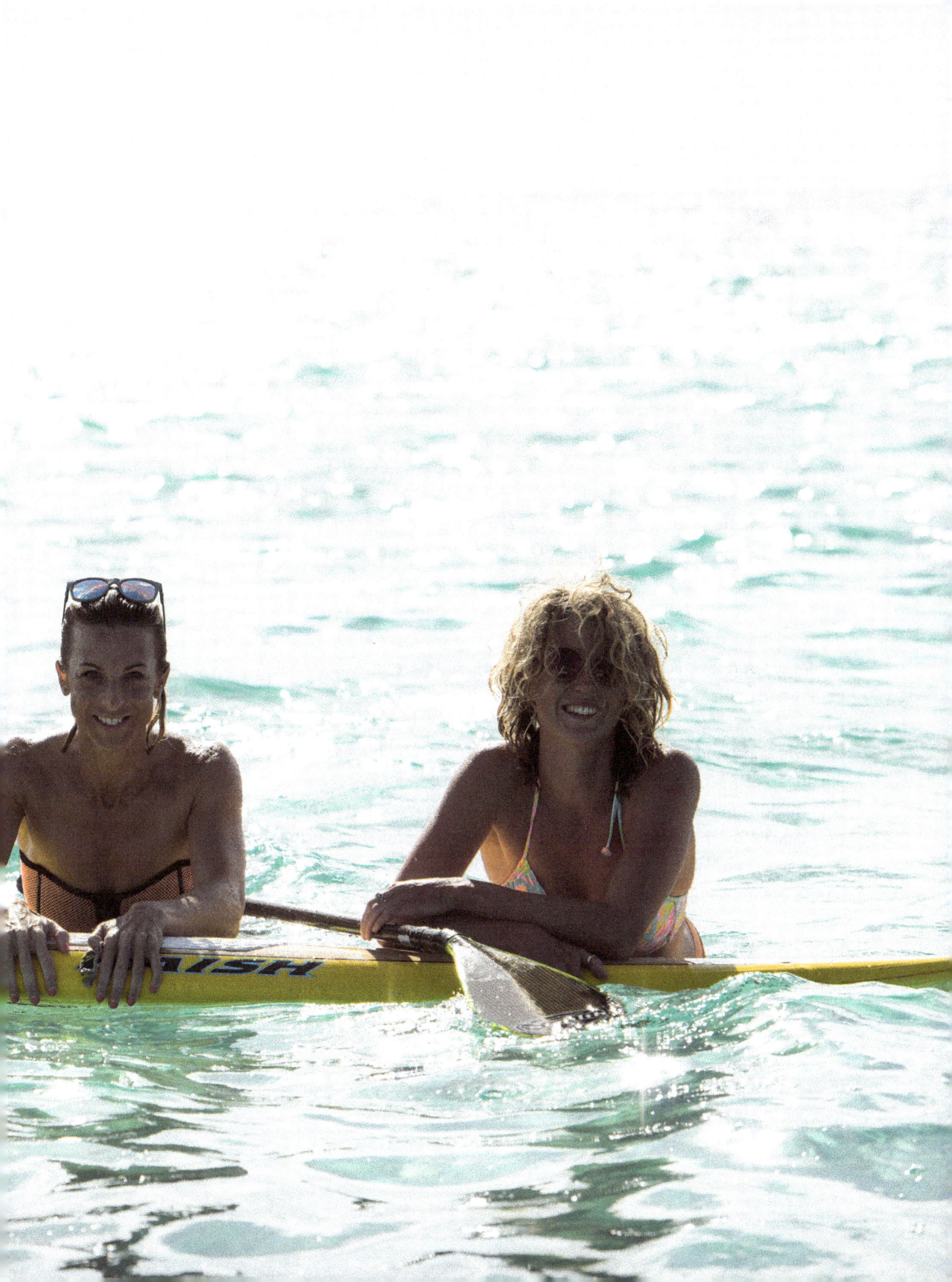

Let's get back to finding your dream team

When it comes to weight loss, fi tness, vitality and overall wellbeing, everyone has the opportunity to create their best body ever and make the most of what they have. It's important to build a team of supporters and a lifestyle that supports this goal seamlessly – rather than crunching healthy aspects into four hours a week.

If you are feeling down, tired or downright stuck in a rut then have a look around at all the people that are doing inspiring things with their lives with less fortune, overcoming major injuries and setbacks and appreciating every day.

Why do we use excuses like not enough time, too busy, need to work, have to be home for the family or I'm not the same as I was when I was younger? Why wait till there is serious injury or a health warning to get your life back in balance? Now is the time and you need to surround yourself with the right positive infl uencers to get things done.

It can really help to get support from key people around you. Be determined and be clear. If you don't ask those you love and your friends for what you need from them, then you can't expect to feel supported. It is human nature for people to test your willpower and want to see how committed you are to your goals.

I'm always inspired by those around us who are open and honest journey to create an amazing life ahead of a serious setback. Hard work, a sense of humour and serious dedication to doing something with life keeps people going and leads to work that inspires others. Hop onto the free Vitality Coach podcast and listen to some inspiring infl uencers that DO things with life, are accountable and never ever give up. It always helps to put things into perspective and remember you ALWAYS have a choice.

Find inspiration and support via podcasts, motivating people, trainers and leaders in your company.

Discover new friends through the new healthy activities you start to do.

When building your dream team of like-minded individuals, remember: they may or may not be your family or close friends, but instead, those that can relate to your goals. These people will lift you up, not try to drag you down.

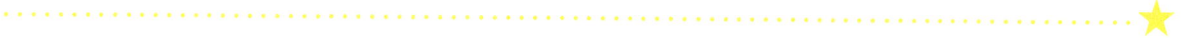
NOTE

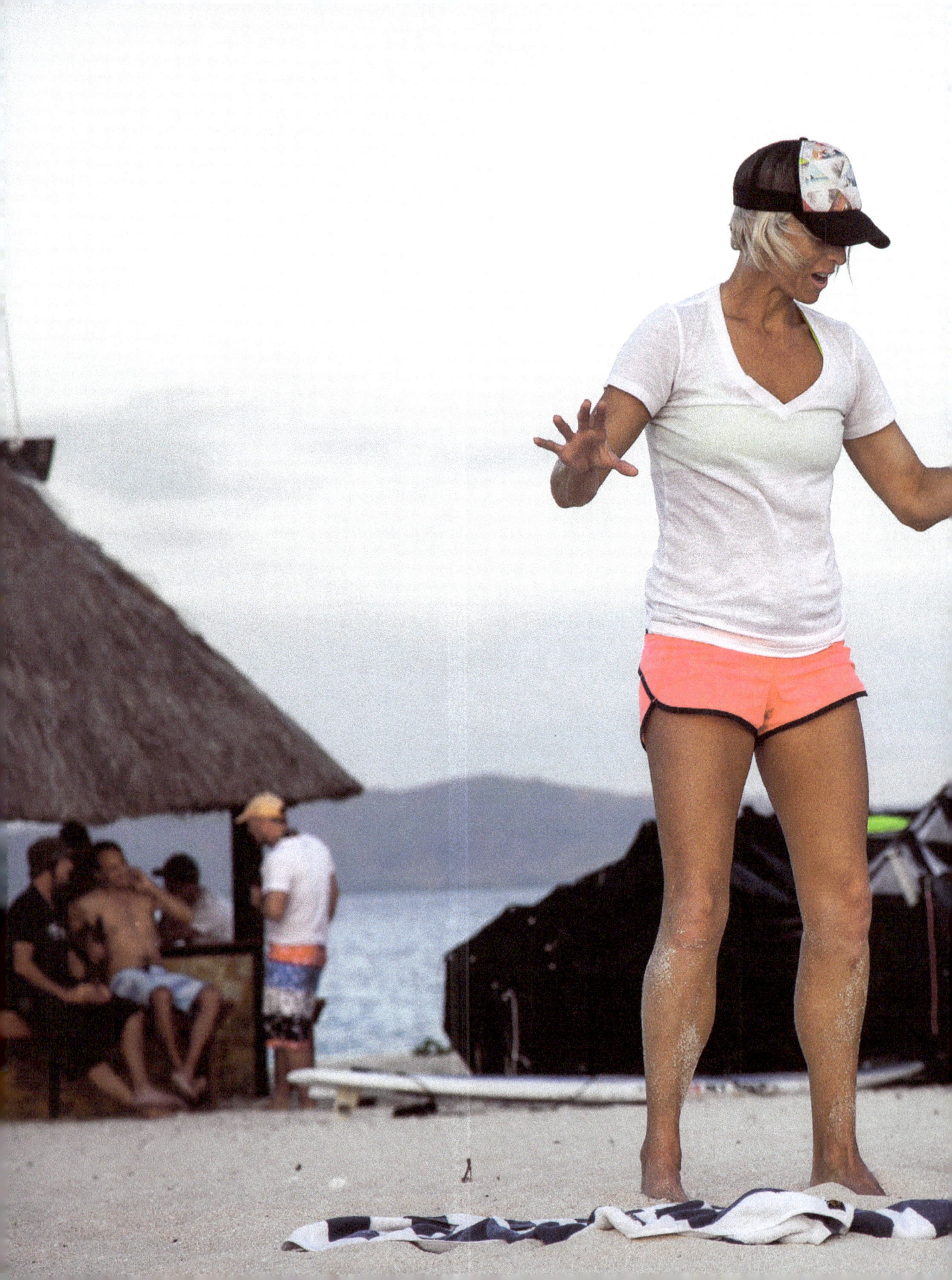

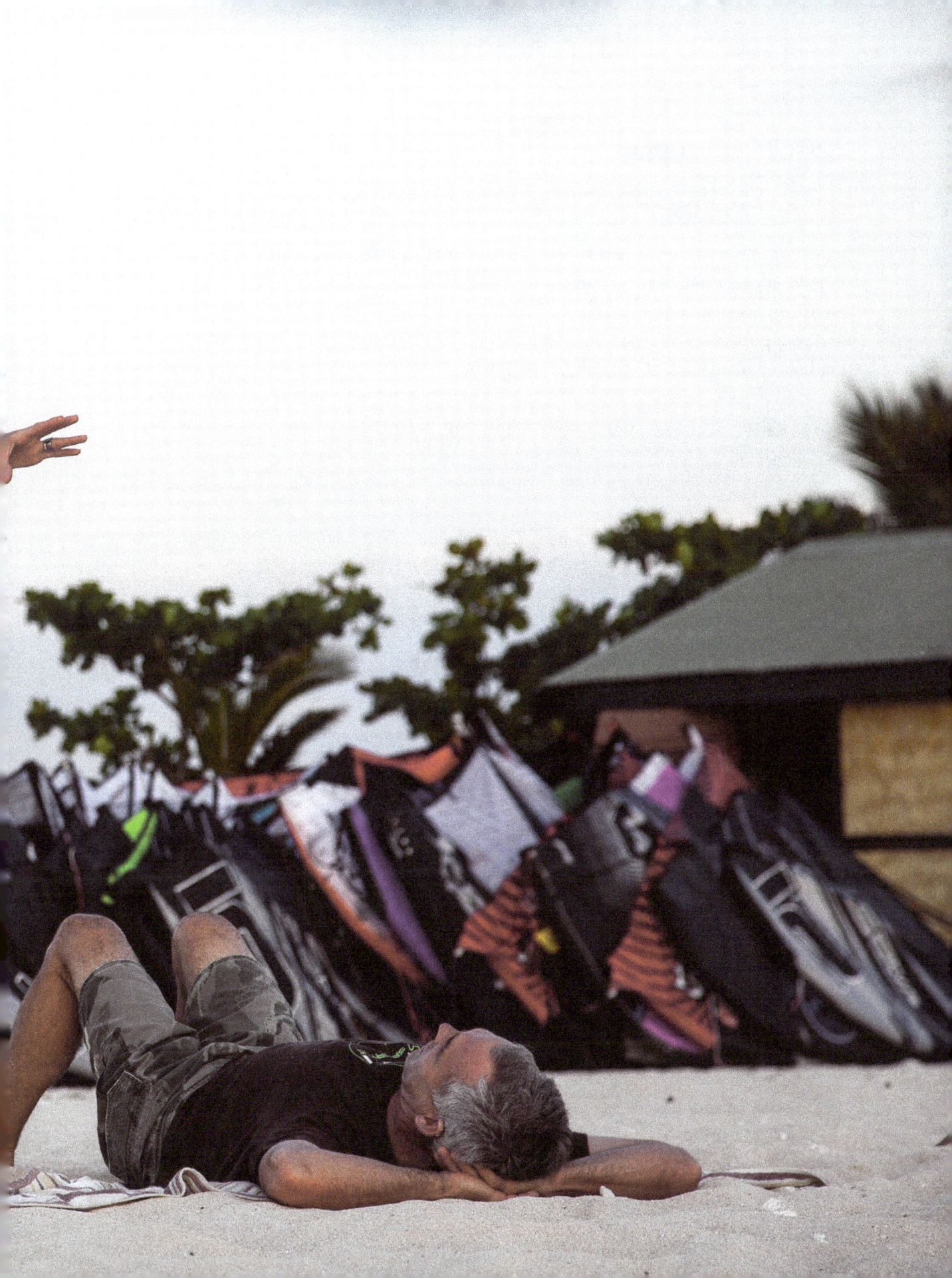

Finding Great Trainer!
Top 10 traits of a great trainer

It's not all about fancy gear and environments – amazing trainers have knowledge and the ability to tailor support and instruction to any environment on any given day. As a consumer you should be asking questions and ensuring you have the best support to suit your needs, budget, goals and your personality. Working out and achieving your personal best is an incredible journey and made even more fun and engaging when you have the best dream team.

Not all trainers are equal, so here is my offi cial top 10 traits checklist to help you identify the best coach!

1. Inspiring
As a client, you must think WOW when you meet your trainer – time and time again.

2. Experienced
Trainers need to know their stuff, be honest about their experience and set rates and standards accordingly.

3. Articulate
Verbal and written communications are a high priority so you can clearly understand what your trainer is telling you.

4. Presentable
Presentation is key to success. Consistently delivering an expert attention to detail means your trainer has pride in what they do and who they are.

5. Professional
Great trainers are professional at all times, as they know that creating a solid and open relationship with clients is key to success – theirs and yours.

6. Organised
Your trainer should be organised by planning ahead and keeping track of programs and information on your behalf. Being on time is also mandatory.

7. Considerate

Preferred trainers understand that life throws curve balls. As professionals, they can assess when the client needs more R&R than a tough session.

8. Knowledgeable

Hand in hand with experience comes knowledge and most importantly, the ability to apply knowledge in any given situation.

9. Adaptive

Not all days are the same, not all clients are the same. The ability to think on their feet, tap into knowledge and experience is a real added value for any trainer.

10. Able to lead by example

By sharing success stories and struggles, your trainer shows you that they practice what they preach, no exceptions.

Dealing with life's little setbacks

Here's the deal in life: you may not have a choice or complete control over a situation or event. However, you can determine your reaction and the outcome for yourself. It all comes down to your mindset.

Twisting your ankle before a big race can be really bad luck – but it does not discount all the hard work you have put in for the weeks leading up to the event. You can always pick up where you left off once your ankle has healed. In other words? Do not give up. Ever!

The universe loves to test our fortitude. Just when we think it s all coming together, something will challenge your status quo. Take a step back to look at the bigger picture and you l soon realise that this is just another situation for you to get through.

Remember: You can create the life you want!

If you're finding it hard to keep your true grit and mental fortitude – or in some cases, you may find it's a lonely road to travel, picking up a healthy new lifestyle when those close to you are still munching fries and burgers – here are some key points to help you through:

Connect: Find like-minded people you can connect with, be inspired by and share ideas with. It might be people you follow on Instagram, at your local yoga studio or gym, friends at a run club, or those you encounter when heading out for a surf.

Review: Keep an eye on the bigger picture. When the going gets tough, step back and look at your master plan. That is your WHY and should remind you not to give up.

Renew: Do something fun! Break your routine, mix it up and get a change of scenery.

Appreciate: Find something positive, no matter how small or inconsequential, to be grateful for. Bring the balance back in to your day by focusing on gratitude and acceptance. Trust me – it works!

The 80/20 rule
Remember the 80/20 rule: stick to your goals and plan 80% of the time. If you head off track don't let that discourage you from the bigger picture. In some ways it will be challenging – but stay relaxed and don't put too much pressure on yourself.

Relax: Take some time out to rest, relax, stock up on healthy foods and do some exercise you enjoy. Be kind to your body in moments of stress and doubt.

Ask for help: Even great coaches need coaches. If you're unsure or feeling stuck, then ask a mentor, trainer, friend, teacher or someone you trust for ideas and support.

Can you list all your procrastinations and put them on paper to see the story you have been telling yourself?

Your Usual Excuses:	Your New Habits:
Example:	Example:

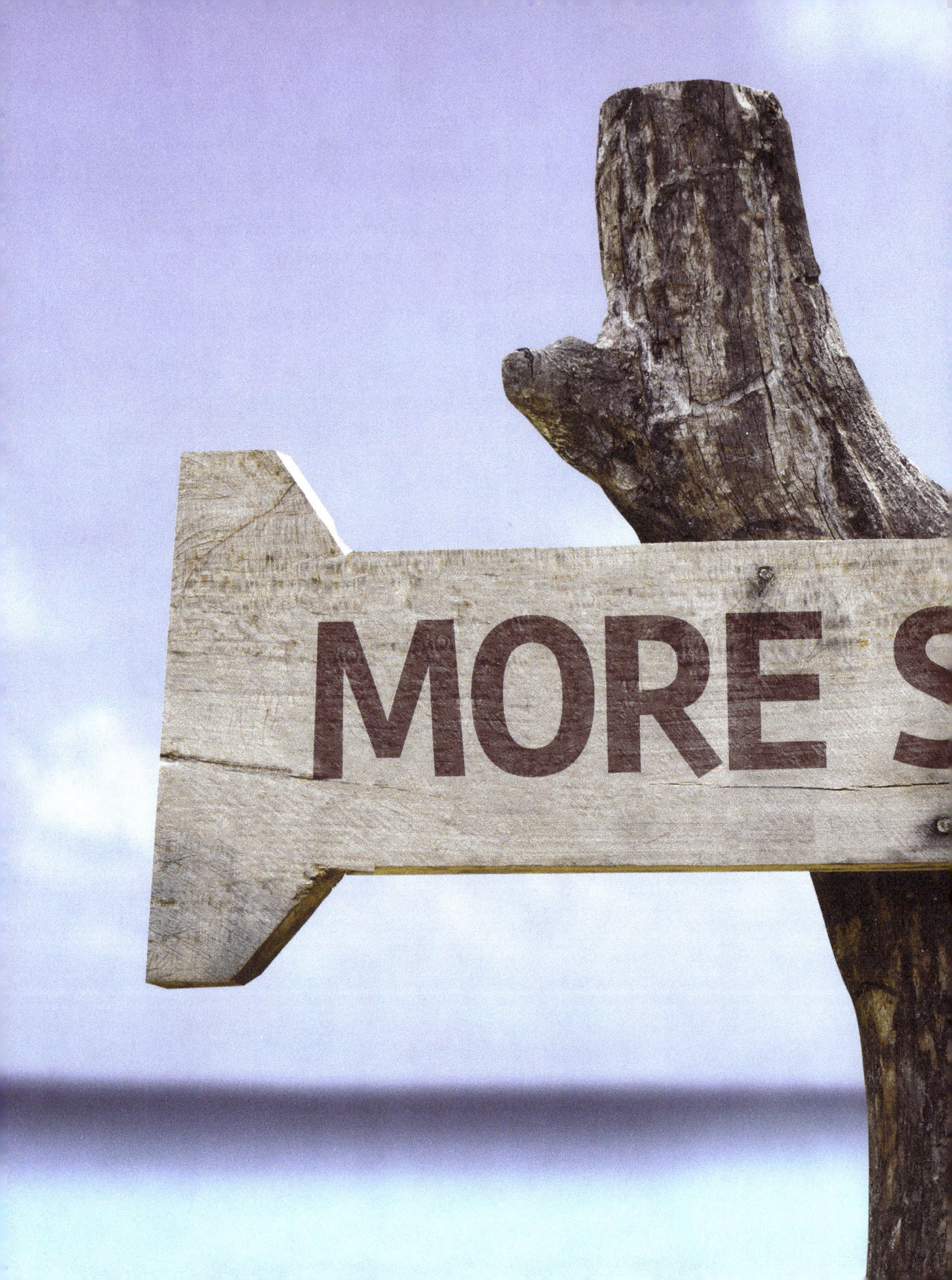
MORE S

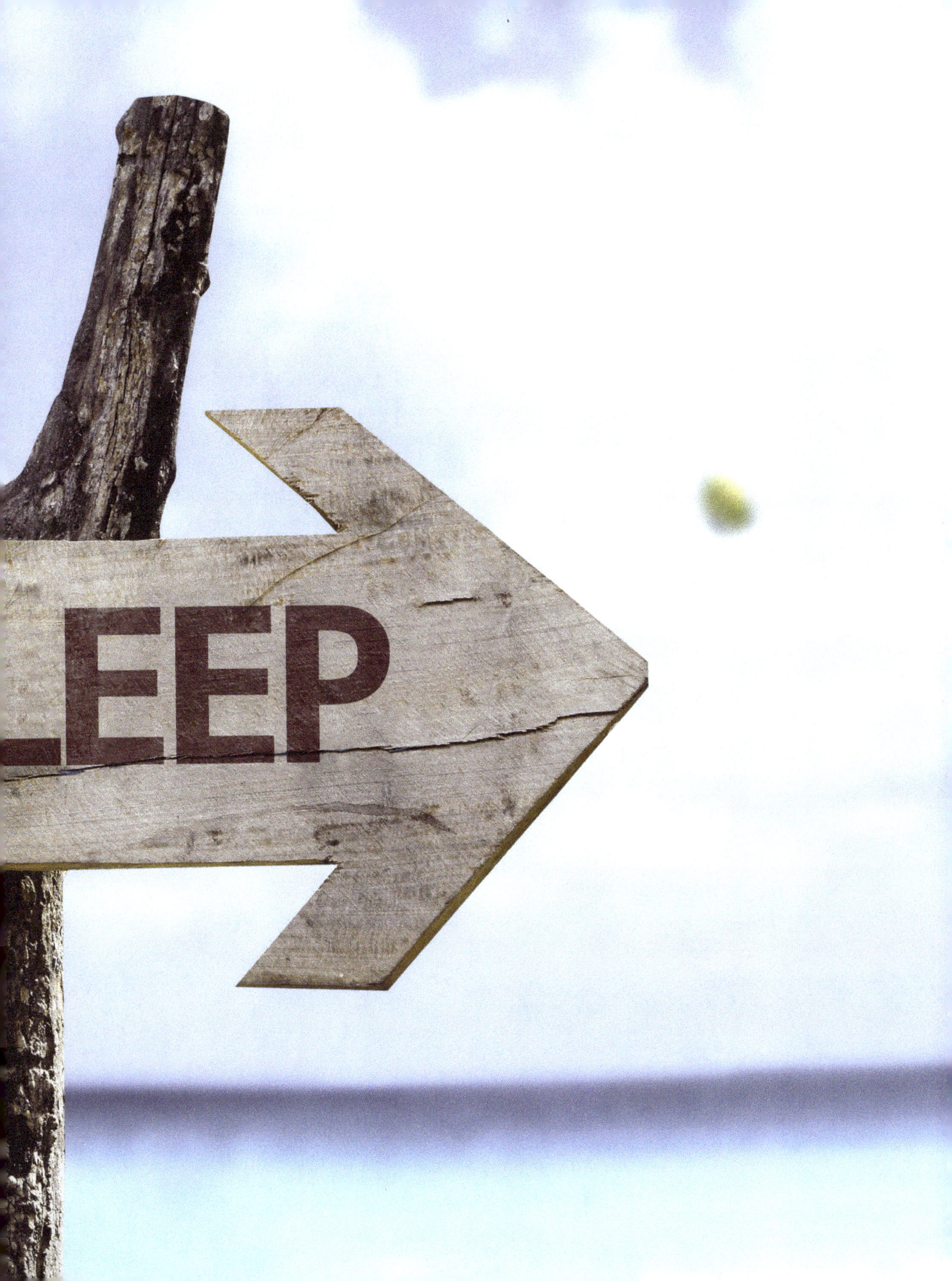

Sleep, glorious sleep!

A lot of emphasis is placed on exercise and diet for general health and wellbeing, but a big part of the wellness picture is often left out: sleep.

Quality sleep is vital to wellbeing. When you are lacking sleep you cannot re-charge, meaning you effectively reduce your levels of optimal health, as well as performance.

Worse still, repeated periods of lack of sleep can play havoc on your hormones, prevent weight loss, reduce memory and mental performance and create dangerous situations, if you are not functioning with 100% attention (such as driving or operating heavy machinery).

Insomnia can be irregular based on circumstances, stress, over-thinking things, over training, a bad diet, the wrong foods before bedtime or even bad lighting and ventilation in the room. The key is ensuring that insomnia and not sleeping through the night does NOT become a pattern.

Sleep patterns are different for everyone: some fall asleep quickly, and others take a while. When you are asleep, your body needs the ability to go into a deeper NREM sleep mode as this is where all the magic happens for cell regeneration, muscle and tissue recovery and recharging of your body battery.

The most common symptoms of insomnia:
★ Difficulty falling asleep
★ Waking up frequently during the night
★ Difficulty returning to sleep
★ Waking up too early in the morning
★ Un-refreshing sleep
★ Daytime sleepiness
★ Difficulty concentrating
★ Irritability
Source: The National Sleep Foundation

A lack of sleep:
★ Reduces your senses.
★ Can affect your memory, mental and physical performance.

★ Is one of the leading causes of road accidents, by people falling asleep at the wheel.

★ Can severely affect your bedroom mojo.

★ Causes excess secretion of the stress hormone, cortisol, which can inhibit weight loss and break down skin collagen, the protein that keeps skin smooth and elastic.

★ Plays havoc on your immune system, increasing your chances of colds, flu and general illnesses as your body is not functioning in its ideal state.

Tips to break the cycle of insomnia:

At night:

★ Avoid TV, illuminated alarm clocks and other digital stimulus in the bedroom.

★ Read a book before you go to sleep, rather than watching television or working late on the computer.

★ Meditate and concentrate on breathing.

★ Channel your thoughts from worry to a place of peace.

★ Create a regular bedtime routine and a regular sleep-wake schedule.

★ Create a restful environment that is dark, cool and comfortable.

★ Play restful music to help you relax.

Keep a diary of things that are on your mind, get them out of your head and on to paper – even if it's a list of things to do for the next day.

During the day:

★ Reduce your caffeine intake and avoid it all together late in the day.

★ Avoid alcohol and nicotine, especially close to bedtime.

★ Do not eat or drink too much of anything within an hour of bedtime.

★ Exercise, but not within three hours before bedtime – make sure you have sufficient time to wind down and relax post-training before heading to bed.

No sleep = depleted batteries

Fit tip:
If you're really struggling with sleep, keep a sleep diary to identify your sleep habits and patterns, so you can share it with your doctor or a specialist. You may find that you start recognising your own patterns and can change some habits. Include foods you eat at nighttime and the time you go to bed as well as get up in the morning.

FRESH AIR + FRESH FOOD +
FRESH PERSPECTIVE =
RECIPE FOR FEELING FANTASTIC

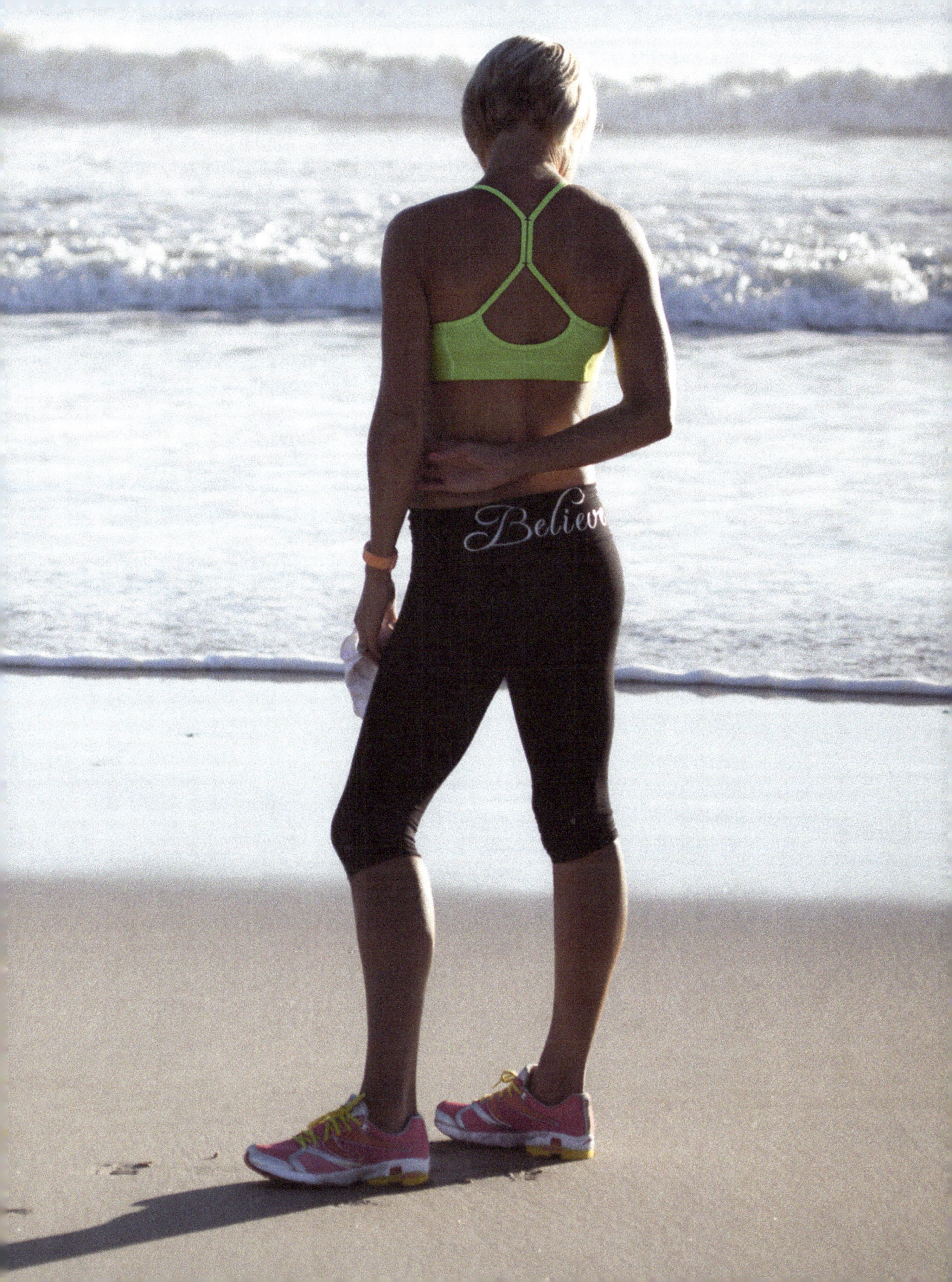

Think of lack of sleep over several nights as your phone never being charged properly from the beginning. This results in the battery life being shorter before it needs to be plugged in and recharged. It works the same for our bodies: if we do not fully recharge our batteries, then we diminish our energy levels, and our ability to handle stress and perform daily tasks.

The importance of balance

Does it ever feel as if life is just speeding by and you're running from one thing to the next, without time to pause and re-group?

Have you lost your sense of humour?

Are you feeling more sensitive or just not feeling quite yourself?

And have you put working out, exercise and general wellbeing at the bottom of the list as you don't have time?

You are not alone!

Despite all the technology we have in our lives that is supposed to save time, it seems like people are more stressed and time poor than ever before.

This is not "news". We all know this is certainly the case; what worries me is that intelligent, savvy people who know what healthy living means, are not taking the most basic steps to slow it down and reboot their hard drive each day.

At a certain point, your body simply says 'NO'. It may be in the form of a cold or flu, a niggling pain or injury, headaches, digestive complaints, skin disorders, insomnia or just the fact you feel exhausted.

By the time it has come to this, it is already a reflection of a low immune system and the cellular impact of stress.

How can you start right now to help deal with stress and help your body cope with daily mental and physical demands?

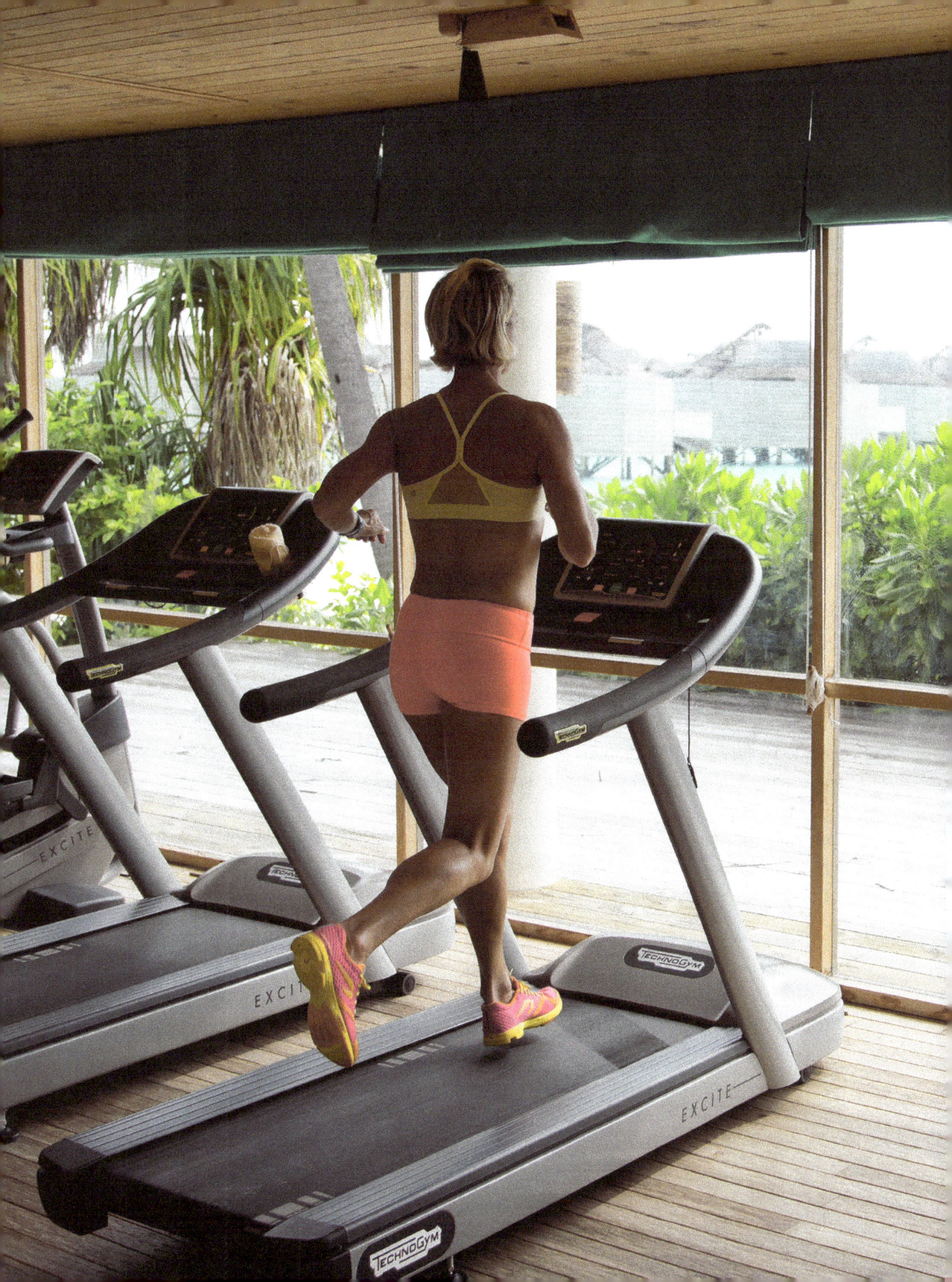

The 1% rule

We should all value our health enough to spend, at the very least, 1% of our 1,440 minutes per day focused on our wellbeing. This means spending just 14 minutes a day on some exercises and functional fitness, stretching, yoga or breathing.

Rather than taking pills, buying potions and worrying about what s wrong, let's start right now…

★ As you are reading this, pull your belly to your spine and adjust your posture.
★ Soften your eyes and keep breathing through your nose.
★ Lift your shoulders to your ears; hold them there as you inhale then exhale and let them drop. Repeat this a couple of times.
★ Be present. Concentrate your breath to reach all areas of your body – from your head to your toes.

Once you've read this, start getting the things that worry you off your mind and onto paper. Letting things circle around your head is not constructive. Writing ideas and worries and things that concern you down helps make them transparent and you can start to see if you should action certain things that warrant your time – or just cross them off completely!

Practice the 1% rule daily. You are a reflection of your approach to health and wellbeing. If you want to be fitter, healthier and happier then YOU alone need to make some changes, by putting some actions into place and practicing some relaxation or exercises.

Commit to mastering 1 exercise per week – practise it daily and by the end of the year you will have 365 exercises you can pull together to create the most incredible set of workouts, combinations and moments bringing mind and body together.

Just commit to 14.4 minutes per day. If you do this for 100 days you will be 100% better off than where you are now.

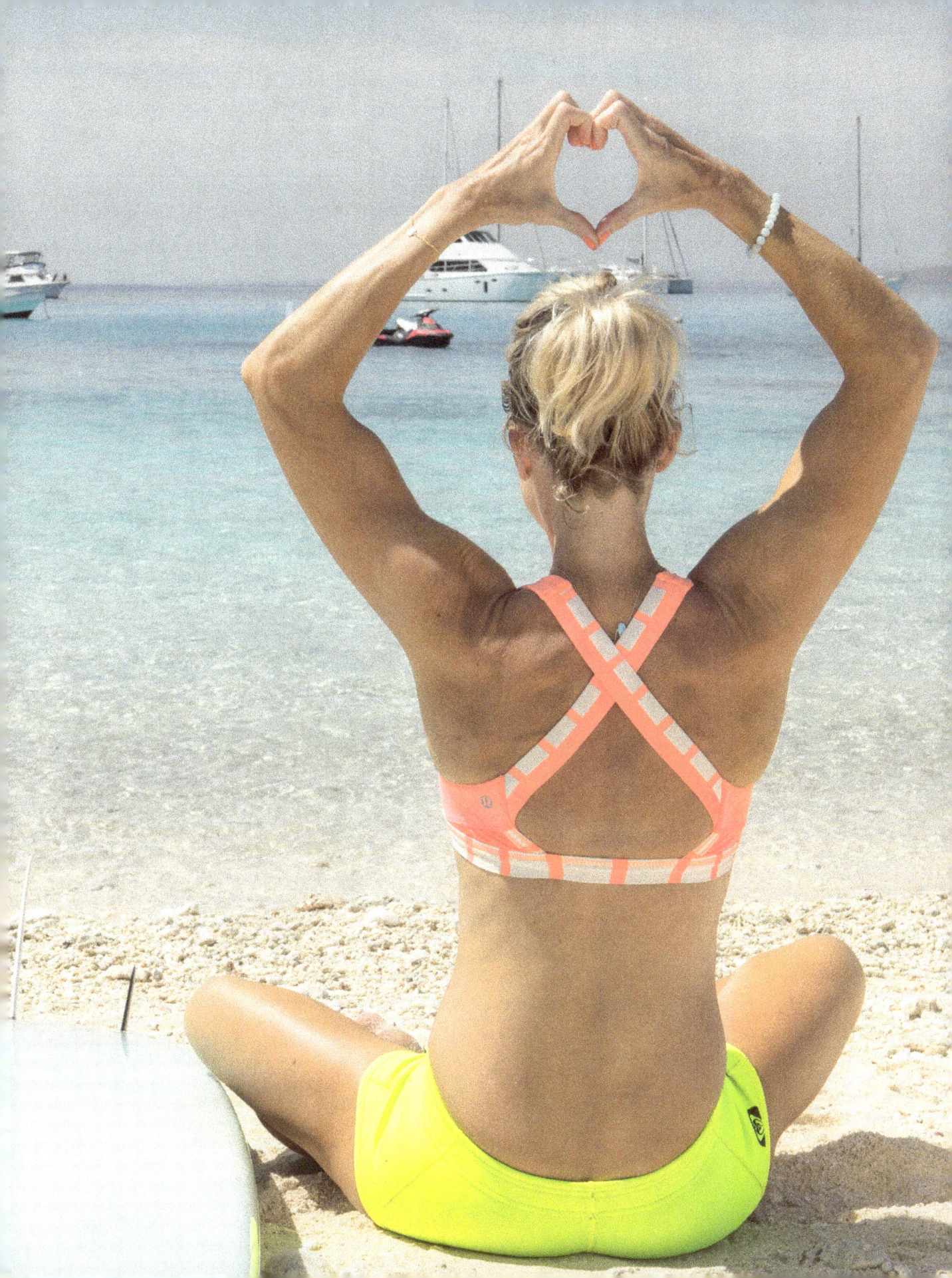

Creating a haven at home

Just as important as having the right attitude and commitment is having the right type of space to encourage you to be the best version of yourself.

Sight: Use lighting to create an environment that is welcoming and soothing. Avoid TV later in the evening and consider reading or just relaxing listening to music as a change of pace. Also consider dimming your lights, using candles and avoiding digital lights in your bedroom.

Sound: Music has the powerful ability to influence your mood. Listen to chilled out sounds for the afternoon and evening to relax and upbeat tempos for the morning. Music has a direct effect on how we feel and sound is one of the strongest sensory systems in our body.

Touch: Consider the pillows and fabrics you use for your bed linen, sofa cushions and throws; these should be natural cottons and soft textures that create a comfortable area to lounge and relax. Booking a regular massage can also do wonders to recharge your body.

Taste: Employ the "fresh is best" philosophy. If you can't grow your own mini herb garden, then shop at farmer's markets, choose fresh food from menus and select ingredients that are more nature based than processed.

Smell: Cook with fresh herbs and spices that activate the sense of smell and let that take you on a culinary journey to different places and cultures. Consider burning organic scented candles in your home or office space that are subtly infused.

Tip:
Spend a few minutes tidying and filing your desk area at the end of each day, and consider storage and display systems at home to show your prized possessions and allow a sense of calm in your home.

Perception: Rid your house and workspace of clutter to allow for a better energy flow and nicer environment, one that can create mental space for your own creativity. By giving yourself peace and quiet to listen to your body, you can create an environment that supports you living to your full potential.

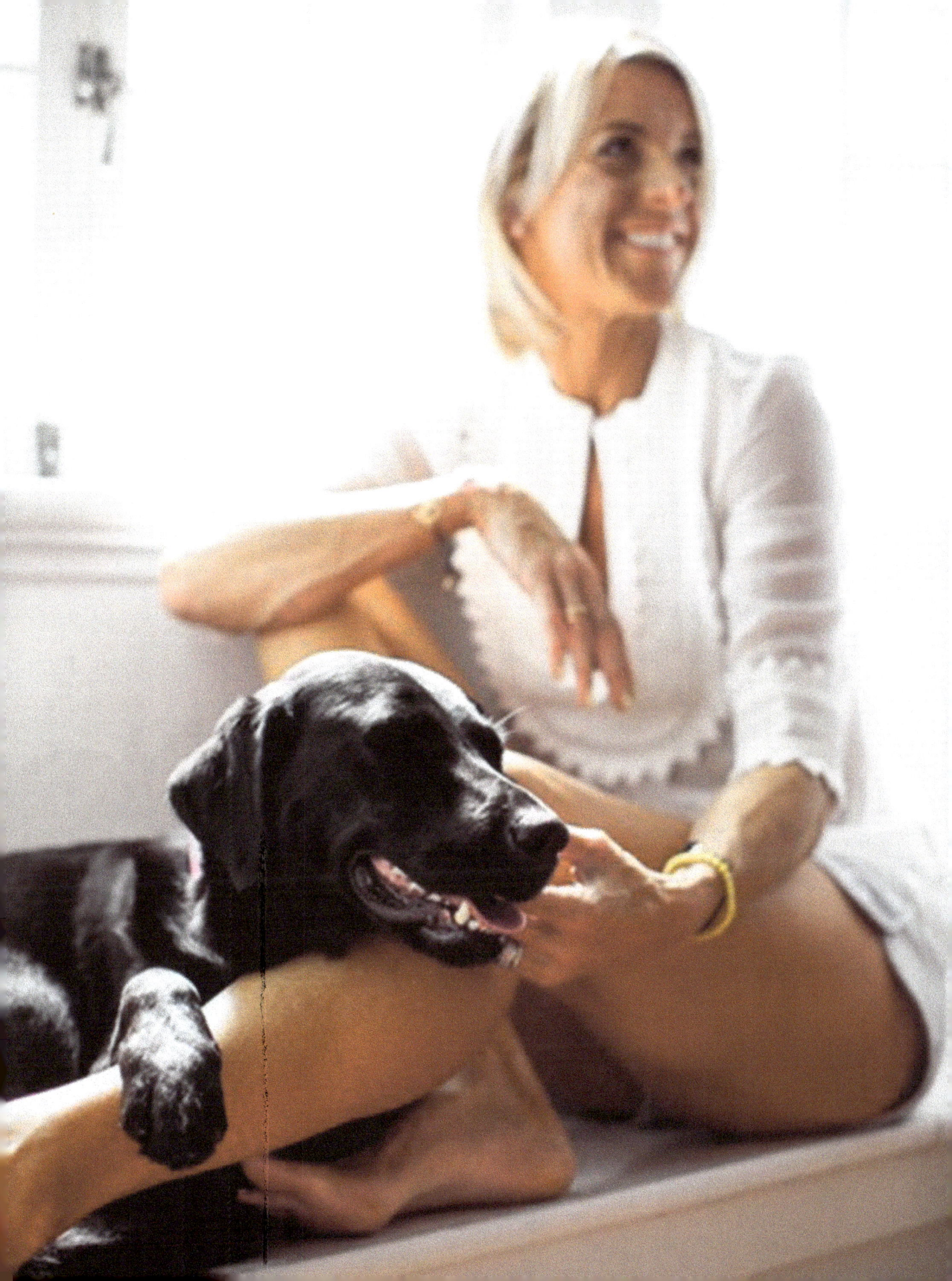

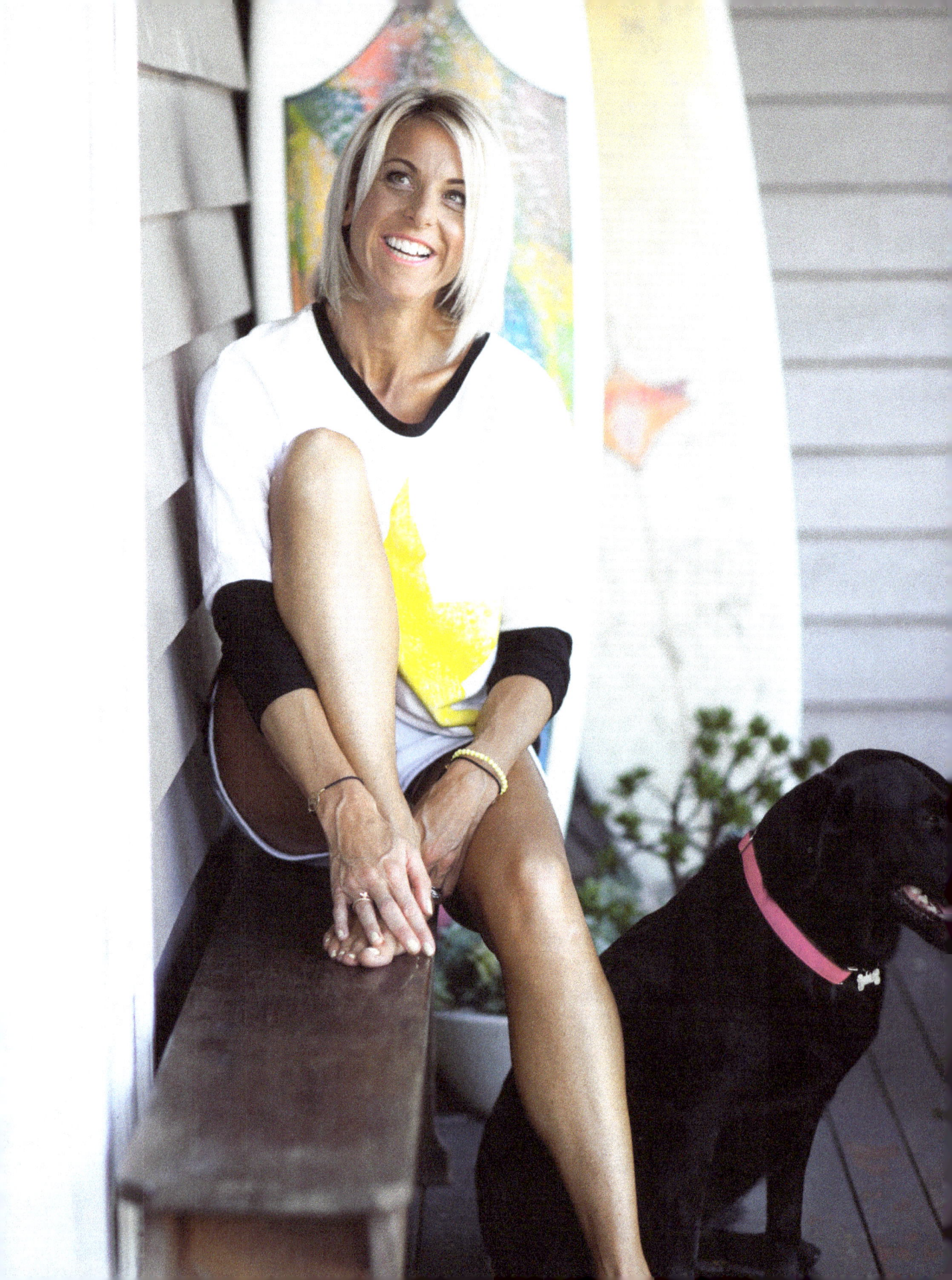

Putting it all into practice

It's important to put **mind over matter** and to keep it simple! These tips will help you live this theory in your daily life:

★ Lace up your shoes and get out the door – regardless of the weather.

★ Don't feel like running? Then just walk!

★ Call a friend and book a gym/yoga/walk/run date.

★ Take your dog for a walk – or offer to walk someone else s who you know doesn't have the time.

★ Share healthy eating habits by cooking for others and becoming their source of inspiration.

★ Bring a salad or delicious healthy dessert if you are a guest at a friend's house.

★ Sign your work team up for a charity run/walk.

★ Play with your kids.

★ Explore the city on foot.

★ Celebrate all that you have rather than focusing on what you can't do.

★ If in doubt, walk it out. Put all your thoughts on the back burner and just go get some fresh air.

★ Visit farmer's markets on the weekends and start reconnecting your taste buds with what real, whole foods taste like.

★ Throw out all the fad diet mixes, elixirs, artificial sweeteners, toxic tonics and anything else with ingredients you can't pronounce, and get back to basics with fresh food and ingredients that are as close as possible to their natural states. Your body will thank you for it!

Remember: Being fit and healthy should not be expensive. It is a mindset, not a 'gym set' way of life that is integrated seamlessly into your day, without too much effort or tuning your life upside down.

Actions speak louder than words, so all the goal setting, planning and wish listing in the world means nothing if you don't start living, sharing and celebrating what you believe!

Make time to let your intuition be heard. If you are forcing decisions or over analysing you are wasting valuable time of *actually living.*

You don't need all the answers at once; just take one step forward and the rest will follow.

"So what now?"

You are on a mission!

Taking full responsibility for yourself is a key pillar for my coaching with clients and is part of my own personal values.

Essentially it's about taking your life off autopilot. Becoming accountable for your actions and knowing that you – you alone, create the life you want.

Being informed and educated on how you can truly reach your potential and live a happy fulfilling life, starts with taking responsibility. There are no quick fixes really – not if you want lasting results. It's all in your mindset.

Remember: you can absolutely create the life you want.
I am living proof of that!

This is just the start of the journey and a small snapshot at some basic tips and tools to get you to the next level of feeling and living your personal best.

I've got loads more on youtube, my blog, podcasts and inspirational quotes on Instagram you can download, read and watch anytime for free. Coming up soon will be the follow up in the Vitality Book series, focusing on the real sweet spot for balance in a busy world, specific mini programs for cycling, running, swimming and also NATURE IS YOUR GYM – one I can't wait to share with you.

As always – I'm an email or a message away. Please let me know what challenges you face and how if any of the elements in this book have helped you rebuild confidence in your own knowledge and rediscover your mojo.

We have just one life, the same hours, minutes, days and months in a year as everyone else. Its really personal choice what we do with this all.

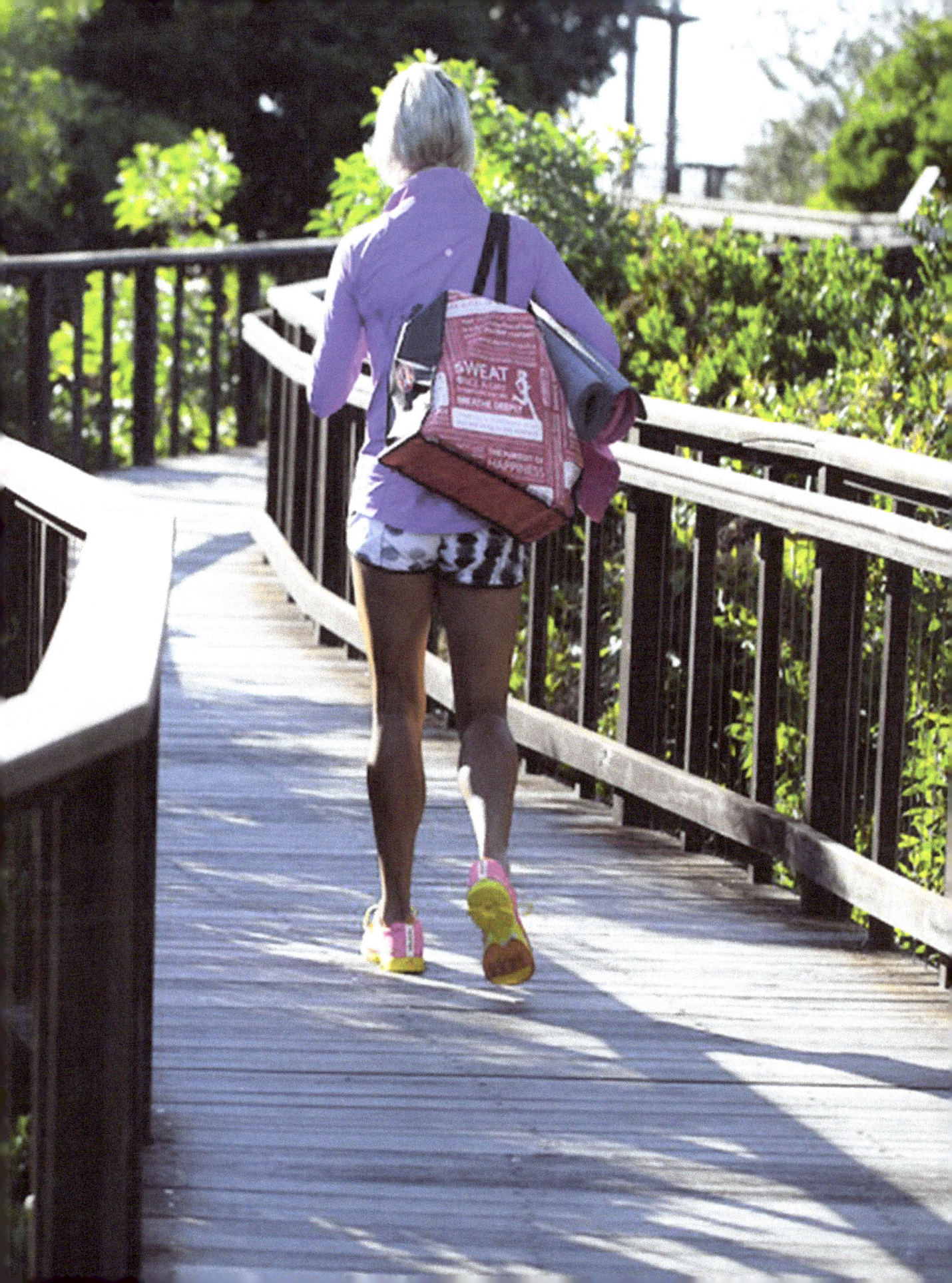

I hope that you're reading this because you're a person that does things with life – you grab opportunities with both hands, work hard, love well and live your life to the max. Just remember to re-group regularly, to take time to calibrate and ensure you're on the path you want, rather than the one you're given.

Can't wait to connect with you and hopefully meet some of you in person on my Vitality Tour.

Health & Happiness
Your Vitality Coach

Nikki

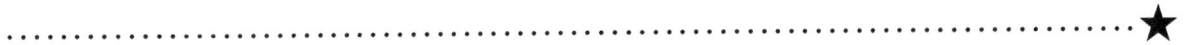

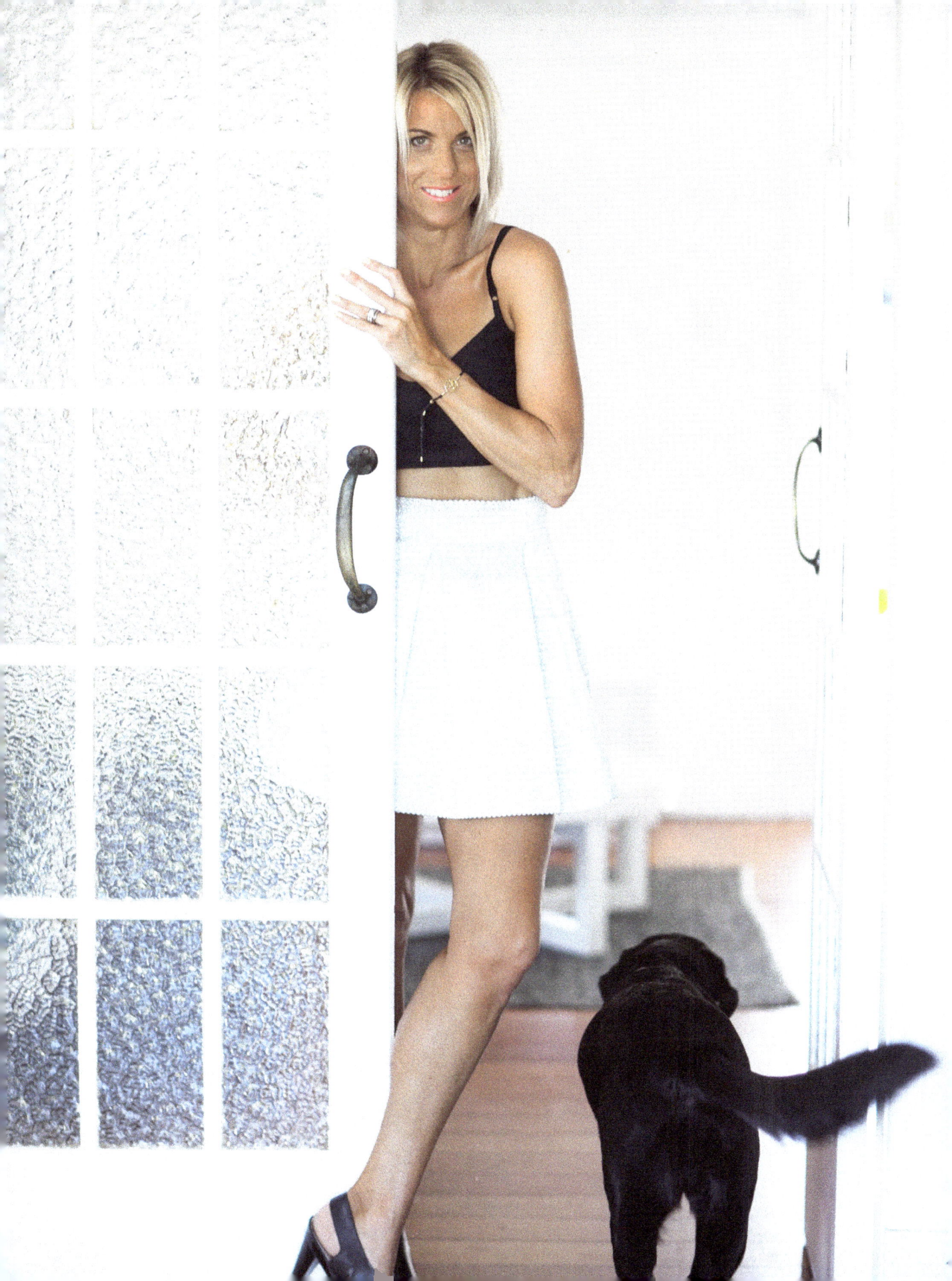

INDEX

www.ingramcontent.com/pod-product-compliance
Lightning Source LLC
Chambersburg PA
CBHW080250030426
42334CB00023BA/2764

9780648261834